Endoscopic Sinus Surgery

New Horizons

Nikhil J. Bhatt, M.D.

Assistant Clinical Professor
Dept. of Otolaryngology
University of Illinois
Eye and Ear Infirmary
Chicago, Illinois

Director
Sherman Laser and Advanced Surgery Center
Sherman Hospital
Elgin, Illinois

SINGULAR PUBLISHING GROUP, INC.
SAN DIEGO • LONDON

Editor: Marjorie Pannell
Assistant Editor: Valerie Garcia
Project Manager: Kent Szadowski
Production Editor: Nikhil Bhatt, M.D.
Designer: Nikhil Bhatt, M.D.

Singular Publishing Group, Inc.
401 West A Street, Suite 325
San Diego, California 92101-7904

Singular Publishing Ltd.
19 Compton Terrace
London N1 2UN, U.K.

e-mail: singpub@mail.cerfnet.com
website: http://www.singpub.com

© 1997 by Singular Publishing Group, Inc.

Produced by Educational Technology Ltd.
Printed in Singapore by Stamford Press Pte Ltd.

All rights, including that of translation reserved. No part of this publication may be reproduced, stored in a retrieval system or transmitted in any form or by any means, electronic, mechanical, recording, or otherwise, without the prior written permission of the publisher.

Library of Congress Cataloging-in-Publication Data

Bhatt, Nikhil J.
    Endoscopic sinus surgery : new horizons / Nikhil J. Bhatt
      p.   cm.
    Includes bibliographical references and index.
    ISBN 1-56593-897-6
    1. Paranasal sinuses—Endoscopic surgery. I. Title.
    [DNLM: 1. Paranasal Sinuses—surgery. 2. Paranasal Sinuses—anatomy & histology.
    3. Surgery, Endoscopic—methods. WV 340 B575e 1997]
RF421.B48 1997
617.5'2—dc21
DNLM/DLC
for Library of Congress   97-20818
                                                                                 CIP

Extreme care has been taken to maintain the accuracy of the information contained in this book. Neither the publisher nor the authors can be held responsible for errors or any consequences arising from the use of the information contained herein.

This book is dedicated
to the memory of my father,
Jashwant Shyam Bhatt,
whose aspirations and ambition for me
culminated in this effort.

Foreword

Functional endoscopic sinus surgery (FESS) represents a major technical advance in the history of sinus surgery. As minimally invasive surgical procedures benefit patients in the broad spectrum of surgical fields, so too has FESS refined the sinus surgical experience.

As in other systems within the head and neck, the anatomy of the sinuses and paranasal sinus regions is complex and varied. Acute and chronic processes render precise anatomical identification more difficult for the surgeon. For these reasons the potential complications spawned from inexact FESS may be significant and even life-threatening.

In 1628 William Harvey stated it best: "I profess to both teach and learn anatomy, not from books, but from dissections, not from the position of philosophy, but from the fabric of nature."

In this spirit, Dr. Bhatt has authored an exquisite clinically oriented text atlas of endoscopic sinus surgery. By correlating surgical endoscopic images with anatomical sections and CT images, precision diagnosis and targeted surgery are masterfully revealed for the learner and expert alike. The beautiful color slides and renditions merit immediate appeal; additional value derives from the many insightful clinical "tricks of the trade" revealed in abundance.

Those practitioners interested in FESS will benefit from not only reading, but *studying* this important contribution.

M. Eugene Tardy, Jr., M.D., F.A.C.S.
President, American Board of Otolaryngology

Professor of Clinical Otolaryngology - Head and Neck Surgery
Director of Division of Head and Neck Plastic Surgery
University of Illinois Medical Center at Chicago
Chicago, Illinois

Professor of Clinical Otolaryngology - Head and Neck Surgery
Indiana University School of Medicine
Indianapolis, Indiana

Preface

Several stalwart individuals have inspired me throughout my career. This book is a culmination of that inspiration. My uncle Dr. J. S. Bhatt, a general practitioner, always insisted, "Be an excellent anatomist, before you be anything else. You should close your eyes and be able to recognize the structures." Dr. S. S. Balge, my Ear, Nose and Throat Professor in India, encouraged me to be bold and curious. "Search and you shall find" was his motto. Dr. Albert Andrews, the pioneer in laser surgery in laryngology, sparked my interest in lasers while I was at the University of Illinois. Dr. Skolnik taught me to be carefully aggressive in surgery. Dr. Soboroff reinforced the importance of learning and relearning anatomy. It was he who awoke in me a desire to teach. This resulted in several courses that I have been giving all over the country and abroad. Finally, I hope I have been able to achieve the finesse in surgery that I always admired in Dr. E. Tardy.

Having been inspired to compile and disseminate the knowledge that I had gathered over the last several years, I was further encouraged by my father, who insisted that I write a book. I am sure he would be proud of the result.

This book could not have been successfully written by me alone. Several people have helped me along the way. The text was mostly written by my wife, Dr. Anjali Bhatt. The ideas are mine, the language is hers. My son, Sameer, has been invaluable in assisting me with the computer enhancements. My daughter Priya, always concerned about my well-being, made sure that I was well rested and refreshed before I embarked on this task every day.

I am extremely appreciative of the patience and dedication of the operating room staff while I spent extra time videotaping the procedures. Dave Pflederer, the hospital photographer, was a great help in some photographic work and in drawing some of the artist's sketches. Valerie Garcia, Nancy Shrake and Lynn Heugh were of great help in typing and proofreading the manuscript. I am grateful for the support of Sherman Hospital's administration, particularly Mr. John Graham, in allowing me to conduct courses and collect material for my book.

Dave Garcia of the University of Illinois was tremendously helpful in preparing sections of cadaveric heads. The laser slides were provided by LaserScope, and I am grateful for their help.

Finally, it was only with the constant encouragement of my family, particularly all my in-laws, friends and colleagues that this book was completed in a timely manner.

I hope all of my readers agree that I have done them proud and this book will achieve the goal that I had in mind: To improve the techniques of endoscopic surgery, resulting in improved patient care.

Acknowledgments

I wish to acknowledge and express thanks to a few colleagues who have made contributions to some of the chapters:

Dr. Dinesh Mehta, for his innovative ideas on minimizing surgical trauma, which led to the creation of Chapters 4 and 6. Dr. Mehta and I have become a team in the last few years, giving courses and presenting scientific exhibits, and during this time and in the course of several visits to Chicago, his discussions and input have been very valuable for this book.

Dr. Donald Kennard, for writing Chapter 2 and spending significant time and effort in helping to set up the CT scans for this book. With his and Dr. Desai's input we won the Academy Award for our scientific exhibit on "Cross-sectional Anatomy for Functional Endoscopic Sinus Surgery...*to simplify a difficult task!*" in 1994. This exhibit became the basis for this book.

Dr. Jack Anon and Dr. Marvin Fried, for adding the latest in technology by providing Chapter 11.

Dr. Stephen Becker, for writing the text and providing photographs for "Technique for Sphenoethmoidectomy." in Chapter 7.

Dr. Ashim Desai, for spending time in preparing photographs and organizing Chapter 2 and last but not least...

Dr. Dharambir Sethi, who not only co-wrote "Endoscopic Pituitary Surgery" in Chapter 10, but whose constant encouragement and help at various stages of writing, printing and publishing was invaluable in the evolution of this book.

Contributors

Dinesh Mehta, M.D.
Vice Chairman and Associate Professor
Dept. of Otolaryngology
Albert Einstein College of Medicine
Bronx, New York

Jack B. Anon, M.D., F.A.C.S.
Associate Clinical Professor
Dept. of Otolaryngology
University of Pittsburgh
Pittsburgh, Pennsylvania

Marvin P. Fried, M.D.
Associate Professor of Otology and Laryngology
Harvard Medical School
Boston, Massachusetts

Chief, Joint Center for Otolaryngology
Beth Israel Deaconess Medical Center
Brigham and Woman's Hospital
Dana Farber Cancer Center
Boston, Massachusetts

Dharambir S. Sethi, F.R.C.S.
Acting Head and Consultant
Dept. of Otolaryngology
Singapore General Hospital
Singapore

Donald Kennard, M.D.
Assistant Clinical Professor
Dept. of Radiology
University of Illinois
Chicago, Illinois

Stephen Becker, M.D.
Clinical Associate Professor
Dept. of Otolaryngology
Northwestern University
Chicago, Illinois

Ashim A. Desai, M.D.
Otolaryngologist
Bombay, India

Contents

1	**Introduction**	**1**
	Correlations of Endoscopic Cadaver Anatomy with CT Endoscopic Findings	2
	Surgical Significance and Surgical Technique	8
2	**Coronal-Sectional Anatomy with CT Section Correlations**	**24**
3	**Regional Surgical Anatomy**	**30**
	Ethmoid Sinus	30
	Maxillary Sinus	36
	Nick's Triangle	39
	Frontal Sinus	42
	Sphenoid Sinus	48
4	**Minimally Invasive Techniques in Endoscopic Sinus Surgery**	**52**
	Principles of Minimally Invasive Surgery	54
	Instruments	56
	Microdebriders	58
	Lasers	66
5	**Surgical Techniques for Turbinates and Anatomical Variants (Group I)**	**70**
	Techniques of Inferior Turbinate Surgery	71
	Middle Meatus Obstructive Syndrome	74
	Middle Meatus Reconstruction	74
6	**Surgical Techniques for Ostiomeatal Unit Obstruction (Group II)**	**84**
	Middle Meatal Antrostomy and Maxillary Ostium Reconstruction	84
	Maxillary Endoscopy	88
	Maxillary Ostium Reconstruction with Microdebrider	95
	Inferior Meatal Antrostomy and Nasoantral Window	102
	Canine Fossa Maxillary Endoscopy	104

7 Endonasal Approach to the Frontal Sinus (Groups III A & B) — 106
- Principles and Technique — 106
- Frontoethmoid Disease (Group III A) — 110
- Revision Endonasal Frontal Sinus Surgery (Group III B) — 114
- Pansinusitis with Polyposis (Group III B) — 120

8 Sphenoid Sinus Surgery (Groups III A & B) — 126
- Technique for Isolated Sphenoid Sinus Disease (Group III A) — 126
- Technique for Sphenoethmoidectomy (Group III B) — 128
- Posterior Ethmoidectomy and Sphenoidotomy (Group III B) — 130
- Pansinusitis with Polyposis (Group III B) — 136
- Revision Sphenoidotomy (Group III A) — 138

9 Minimally Invasive Techniques in Pediatric Sinus Diseases — 140

10 Adjuvant Procedures — 148
- Endoscopic Pituitary Surgery — 148
- Dacryocystorhinostomy—Primary and Revision — 154
- Orbital Decompression — 162
- Osteoma — 164

11 Computer Guided Endoscopic Sinus Surgery — 167

References — 171

Index — 173

Sections are color-coded for easy reference.

Endoscopic Sinus Surgery

New Horizons

1
INTRODUCTION

The essence of being a good surgeon is to be a good anatomist. A thorough knowledge of all anatomical configurations and variations equips a surgeon with confidence in his or her ability, an anticipation of what findings to expect and the ability to deal with problems. This is what makes a good surgeon.

It is also an established fact that the anatomy of the paranasal sinuses is the most varied of all the anatomy in the entire body. It is hence very important to be cognizant of all the variations that can occur.

Having performed hundreds of cadaveric dissections and over a thousand endoscopic sinus surgical cases, I have come to the conclusion that the best way to approach a sinus surgically is to compare my knowledge of anatomy with CT scan anatomy presurgically in every case. The two sets of information should be correlated at every step of the endoscopic procedure.

This book attempts to integrate the anatomy, CT scan findings and endoscopic evaluation, and to point out the surgical significance of the knowledge gained from this integration.

I believe that this is the first publication to present such an extensive correlative study of all of the sinuses and to demonstrate its use in the improvement and perfection of surgical techniques. Numerous cadaveric dissection pictures show the salient anatomy. The CT scans demonstrate the same features in patients, and the endoscopic evaluation photographs lead us to the surgical steps. I hope that this book will be a guide to all sinus surgeons in perfecting endoscopic sinus surgery techniques.

The first six pages are a comprehensive look at the most critical and important macroscopic and endoscopic anatomy and CT scan sections. These are followed by standard endoscopic sinus surgical steps that are correlated with these sections.

This book illustrates live surgical procedures in step-by-step continuity. I have used computer-enhanced technology to stress the salient anatomical and surgical features. I hope that this will contribute to improved patient care.

Correlations of Endoscopic Cadaver Anatomy with CT Endoscopic Findings

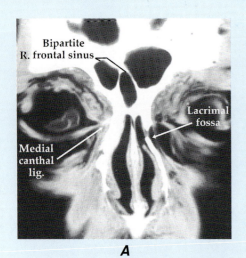

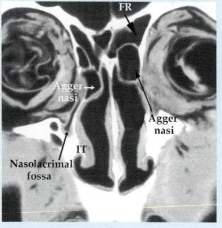

Coronal views at the level of the nasion and 1 cm posterior to it. Note the well-developed agger nasi cells.

A

B

LEVELS OF SECTIONS:

A B C D E F G H

A B C D E F G H

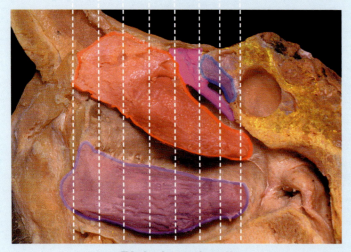

Right lateral wall

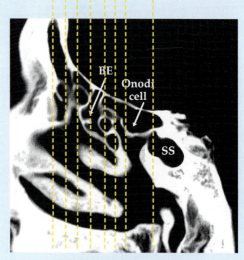

Right lateral wall

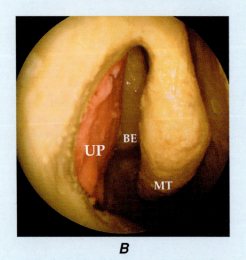

B

Note that the uncinate process and its anterior merge with the firm bony ridge, which is the ascending (frontal) process of the maxilla.

Recognize the agger nasi cell in spite of the absence of the bulge.

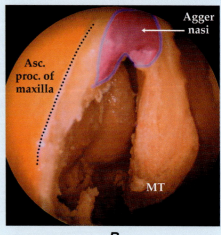

B

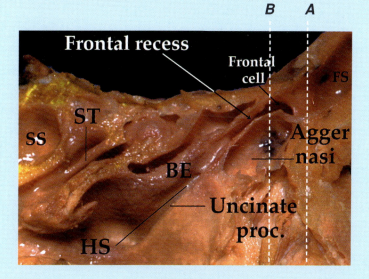

Left lateral wall

Section A

The first section is at the level of the nasion. Here we can see:
- The frontal sinus.
- The ascending (frontal) process of the maxilla.

On the CT section, we also see:
- Part of the nasal bones.
- The medial canthal ligament.
- The lacrimal fossa.
- The anterior nasal septum—note its position.

Sagittal Section

This section demonstrates the relationship of:
- The agger nasi to the frontal recess.
- The optic nerve to the Onodi cell.
- The frontal cell is just above the frontal recess.

Sagittal reconstruction can be done from axial or coronal acquisitions.

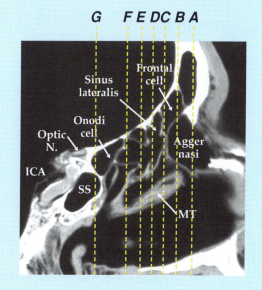

Section B

This section is 1 cm posterior to the nasion. It is the anteriormost section through the inferior nasal turbinate. Note the following:
- The agger nasi cell is adjacent to the anterior lamina papyracea.
- The upper third of the uncinate process forms the medial wall of the agger nasi cell.
- The frontal recess is superior to the agger nasi.
- The section cuts through the nasolacrimal fossa.

On the CT sections, evaluate the position of the nasal septum.

3

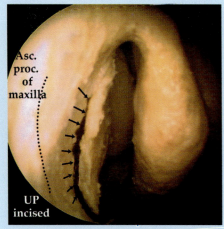

Asc. proc. of maxilla

UP incised

C

This CT section shows the uncinate process and its attachment to the middle turbinate medially and to the lamina papyracea laterally.

Note the space between the uncinate process and the lamina papyracea.

- Incise the uncinate process just below the attachment of the middle turbinate.
- Medialize the UP.
- Separate the UP from the lamina papyracea.
- Define the ethmoid infundibulum.

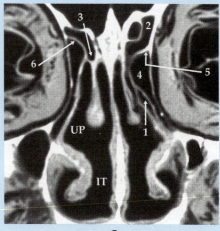

C

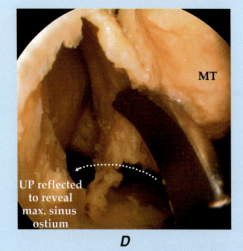

MT

UP reflected to reveal max. sinus ostium

D

A B C DE FG H

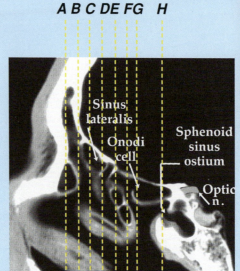

Sinus lateralis
Onodi cell
Sphenoid sinus ostium
Optic n.

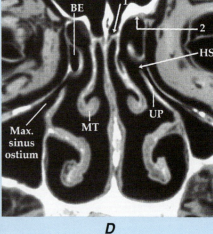

BE
Max. sinus ostium
MT
HS
UP

D

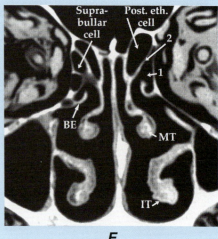

BE
MT
Max. sinus ostium
Resection of medial bullar wall

E

In this section, observe the ethmoid bulla and the number of suprabullar cells. On the right, well-developed bullar and suprabullar cells are present. On the left, they are absent.

The bulla is perforated at its anteroinferior medial quadrant. By staying medial and inferior, we can avoid injury to the orbit.

Suprabullar cell
Post. eth. cell
BE
MT
IT

E

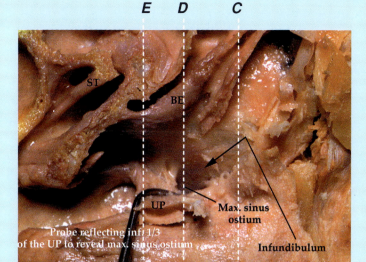

Left lateral wall

Section C

- Note the course of the uncinate process.
- Observe the position of the fovea ethmoidalis bilaterally. The left is higher.
- Study the relationship of the nasal septum to the middle turbinate and to the uncinate process.

Section D

This section is through the ostiomeatal unit.
- Note that the right ethmoid bulla is pneumatized and the left is hypoplastic.

Sagittal Section

- Note the relationship of the agger nasi to the frontal recess.
- Observe the relationship of the frontal recess to the sinus lateralis.
- Note the oblique and horizontal segments of the basal lamella of the middle turbinate.

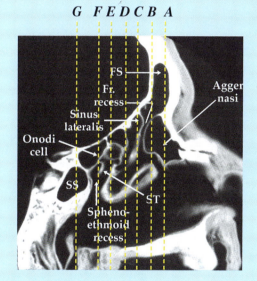

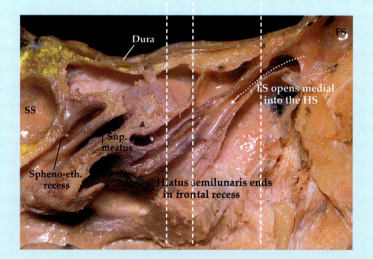

Section E

This section is through the posterior aspect of the uncinate process.
- Note the vertical and oblique attachments of the basal lamella of the middle turbinate to the lamina papyracea and the lateral wall of the nose.

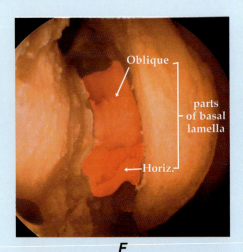

CT section *F* shows:
The oblique attachment of the middle turbinate.
1 = Superior turbinate.
2 = Posterior ethmoid cell.

In this section we can identify the oblique and horizontal parts of the basal lamella. It is quite common to injure the horizontal part during identification of the posterior ethmoid cells.

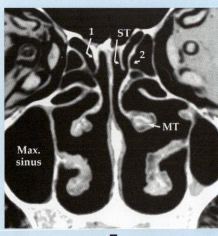

F

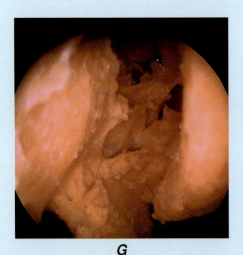

CT section *G* shows:
1 = Posterior conchal cell.
2 = Superior turbinate.
3 = Horizontal attachment of the middle turbinate.
Also seen are the posterior ethmoid cells.

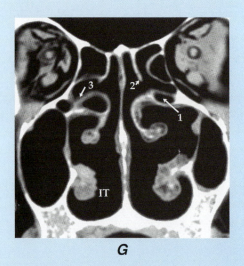

G

The sphenoid sinuses are smaller than usual. Lateral to them are the Onodi cells, which are part of the posterior ethmoid group.

Surgical significance: The optic nerve usually lies in the wall of the Onodi cell when it is present. Hence, it is more liable to injury when dissection is done from anterior to posterior—i.e., when an attempt is made to enter the sphenoid through the posterior ethmoid cells.

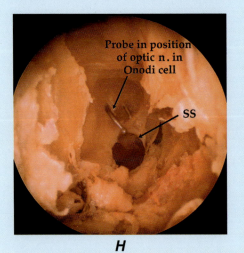

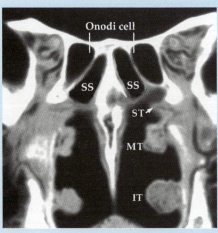

H

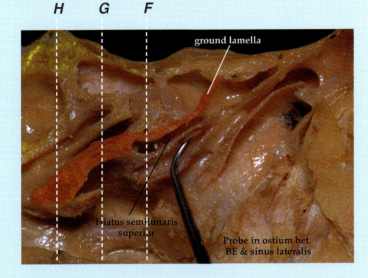

Left lateral wall

Section F

- The superior turbinate arises at the junction of the lamina cribrosa and the fovea ethmoidalis.
- The posterior ethmoid air cell is superior to the horizontal attachment of the left middle nasal turbinate.

Section G

- Note the air cell in the horizontal attachments of both middle turbinates (posterior conchal cell). Also seen in section *F*.
- Posterior ethmoid cells are lateral to both superior turbinates.

The left ethmoid bulla is poorly developed. Though it shows some pneumatization, it lacks definition on the CT section. Correlate with CT section *D*.

In the image on the right, the sinus lateralis is well pneumatized. In such a case, the bulla opens into it.

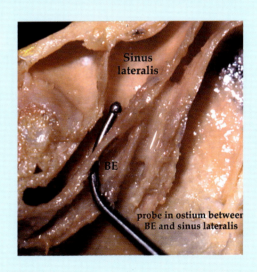

Section H

This section is through the part immediately anterior to the nasal choana.
- The Onodi cell is the posteriormost ethmoid air cell.
- Note the relation of the Onodi cell to the optic nerve.
- The sphenoid sinus remains anteromedial to the Onodi cells.

Surgical Significance and Surgical Technique

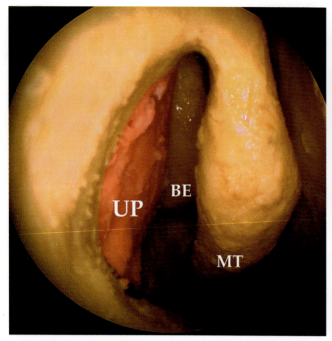 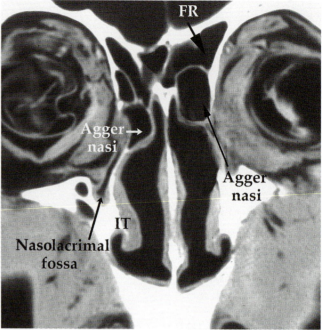

First endoscopic view
Note:
- The size and shape of the middle turbinate.
- The anterior aspect of the uncinate process where it merges with the firm bony ridge—the ascending process of the maxilla.

Look at the junction of this ridge and the middle turbinate attachment:
- Is there any visible bulge?
- Is the vertical lamella of the MT visible?

Look for two bony prominences:
- Uncinate process.
- Bulla ethmoidalis.

Can you see them clearly?

CT section at the level just anterior to the MT
Identify:
- Agger cells.
- Nasolacrimal fossa.
- Frontal recess.
- Position of nasal septum.
  (Anterior septal deviation makes the surgical approach to the agger nasi and frontal recess difficult.)
- At this level, one can see the anterior aspect of the inferior turbinate.

Surgical significance:
- Agger cells may remain hidden and may not make a good bulge. Identification of agger cells during surgery is very important to avoid persistent disease or postoperative recurrence. To identify the agger cells, one must first look at the CT section taken at the level just anterior to the middle turbinate.
- The vertical lamella of the middle turbinate is attached to the lamina cribrosa of the cribriform plate. Forceful medial displacement of the middle turbinate during surgery to expose the ostiomeatal unit area can lead to fracture of the cribriform plate. This can cause two problems:
  1. CSF rhinorrhea.
  2. Loss of anterior stability of the middle turbinate, causing it to flip-flop and subsequently resulting in postoperative lateralization and adhesions.

  To avoid this:
  1. Identify and correct the anterior superior nasal septal deviations.
  2. Perform a modified turbinotomy to facilitate the middle meatus exposure.
  3. Gently compress the middle turbinate medially. This can be accomplished with a freer.

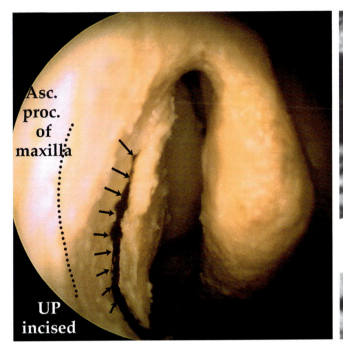
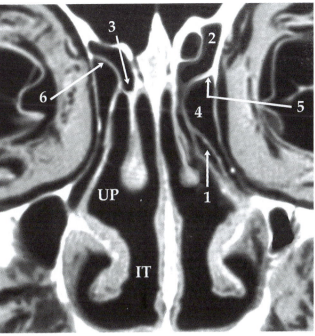

Incision site
- Identify the firm bony ridge—the ascending process of the maxilla.
- Feel the free edge of the uncinate process. Gentle compression gives the feel of the resilience and overhang.
- Look at the CT scan and confirm the presence of lacrimal and/or agger cells.
- Incise from superior to inferior 3 to 5 mm posterior to the ascending process of the maxilla.
- Insert the tip of the sickle knife into the uncinate process just below its attachment to the middle turbinate.

CT section 2 cm posterior to the nasion
1 = Pneumatized uncinate process.
2 = Sinus lateralis.
3 = Attachment of the uncinate process to the MT.
4 = Agger nasi.
5,6 = Attachments of the uncinate process to the lamina papyracea.

The presence of lacrimal and/or agger cells helps to separate the uncinate process from the lamina papyracea, especially at the upper third of its segment. Careful study of CT scans from nasion to midorbital plane will reveal the number, size, and shape of the anterior ethmoid cells; the uncinate process; and the orbital plate (lamina papyracea).

Surgical significance:
- A pneumatized uncinate process should not be mistaken for the bulla ethmoidalis or for a duplicated middle turbinate. In the case of a pneumatized uncinate process, an inadequate incision can lead to problems. The incision leads to the space inside the uncinate process. The lateral wall of the pneumatized uncinate process needs to be resected so we can enter the ethmoid infundibulum.
- If the incision is too close to the free edge of the uncinate process, the anteriormost ethmoid cells may be missed.
- If the incision is too close to the ascending process of the maxilla, the thickness of the bone may cause difficulty.
- At times, the uncinate process merges with the orbital plate, so if the incision is too deep or too high, it is possible to enter the orbit.
- In cases where the anterior ethmoid cells are scarce or absent, the uncinate process and lamina papyracea are almost in apposition to or adherent to one another. In such cases, an incision over the uncinate process can enter the orbit. Reverse elevation of the uncinate process reduces the risk of orbital injury (described later). All cases should therefore be evaluated with presurgical coronal CT scans.

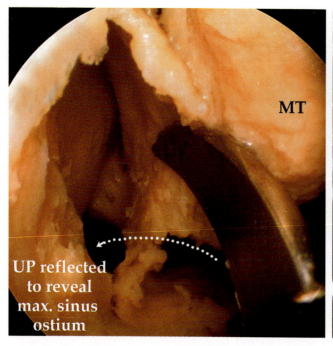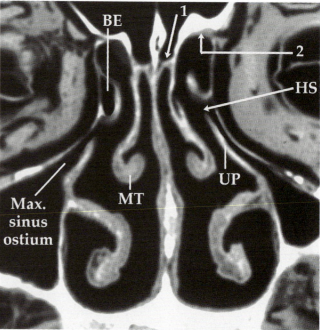

Infundibulotomy
- While doing the uncinectomy, carry the incision downward in a gentle motion.
- Only the tip of the sickle knife should be engaged in the uncinate plate.
- Rotate the knife tip and its handle medially to separate the uncinate plate from its lateral attachments.
- By medializing the inferior third of the uncinate process, one should be able to visualize the ethmoid infundibulum.

CT section through the ostiomeatal unit
The unit is composed of the middle meatus, the maxillary sinus ostium, and the anterior ethmoid. Note that the right ethmoid bulla is pneumatized and the left is hypoplastic. Identify the vertical segment of the basal lamella of the middle turbinate and its attachment to the cribriform plate.
Observe:
1 = Cribriform plate.
2 = Fovea ethmoidalis.
Note the unequal height of the fovea. The left is higher. Evaluate the ethmoid infundibulum for obstruction.

Surgical significance:
- To avoid injury to the orbit or uneven tearing of the mucosa and to identify the maxillary sinus ostium, feel the free edge of the uncinate process and then feel the ascending process of the maxilla, which is the first bony ridge seen and felt in front of the middle turbinate on the lateral wall of the nose.
- The incision is generally placed 4 to 5 mm posterior to the ascending process of the maxilla. Prior to making the incision, feel the recess behind the free border of the uncinate process with a curved ball probe. A to-and-fro motion will give an impression of the condition of the uncinate process. Generally, the uncinate process is quite resilient, and moving its posterior free border allows us to understand its arrangement. Prior to its resection, separate the uncinate process from the lamina papyracea fully. Medialize the uncinate process to expose the infundibulum.
- The maxillary sinus ostium should be reconstructed prior to resection of the agger nasi cells and frontal recess. The reasons for doing this are: (1) The inferior third of the uncinate process serves as an excellent landmark for the maxillary sinus ostium. (2) If the maxillary sinus ostium is kept in view while the frontal recess surgery is performed, it gives good depth perception. (3) Injury to the lamina papyracea is reduced if the maxillary sinus ostium is reconstructed first.

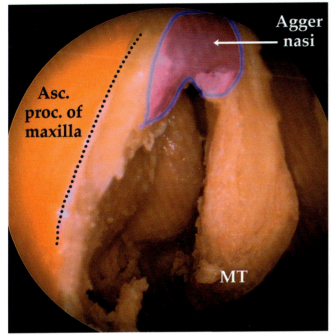 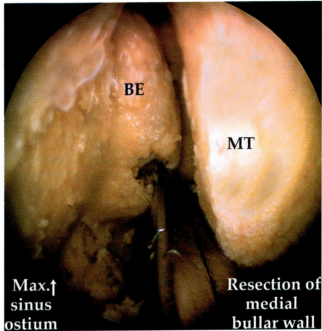

Uncinectomy

As the photograph shows, the upper part of the uncinate process has two attachments—laterally to the lamina papyracea and medially to the middle turbinate. These attachments and their mucosal integrity should be preserved during the uncinectomy. This can be accomplished with a sharp, well-defined incision through both mucosal layers and the uncinate plate just below these attachments. Then, the incision is carried down further.

Approach to the bulla
- The bulla is perforated at its anteroinferior medial quadrant. By staying medial and inferior, one can avoid injury to the orbit.
- Perforate the bullar cell with small straight forceps.
- Insert one jaw of the forceps into the cell, keeping the second jaw outside of the cell.
- Grasp a small part of the medial wall at its most anteroinferior extent. Remove the segment with a gentle medial rotation.
- When the bulla is hypoplastic, it is safer to enter it with a No. 7 Frazier suction. Once the bullar cell is opened, perform sounding to accurately assess its boundaries prior to its resection.

Surgical significance:
- While performing the uncinectomy, resect the upper part with care and leave a small portion as a landmark for superior dissection in the region of the frontal recess. In our experience, the largest number of frontal sinus ostia remain posterior, medial, and superior to the upper attachment of the uncinate process.
- To prevent destruction of the landmark or compromise of the frontal recess, the uppermost portion of the uncinate process should not be crushed.
- When the bulla ethmoidalis is small, it is best to enter the anteroinferior and medial part to avoid injury to the lamina papyracea. Prior to entry into the bulla, the maxillary sinus ostium must be identified. This helps in localizing the ostium.
- Following the anterior wall of the bulla leads to the frontal recess and anterior ethmoid artery crest. The artery is usually posterior to the crest, and the opening of the frontal sinus is anterior to the crest.

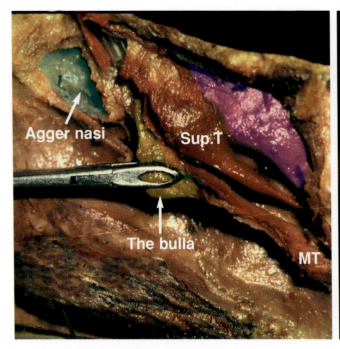
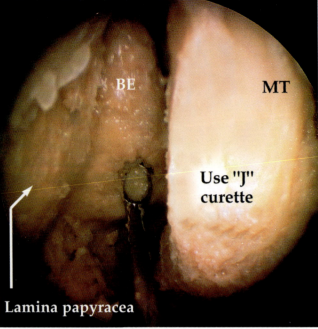

Resection of the medial bullar wall
- Use a small-jaw straight forceps.
- Keep the forceps parallel to the nasal floor.
- Introduce one jaw of the forceps into the anteroinferior wall of the bulla.
- Keep the second jaw medial to the medial wall.
- Control the depth of penetration into the bulla.
- Take a small bite.
- Rotate the forceps clockwise while resecting the bullar wall on the right nasal wall. On the left side rotate counterclockwise.

Defining the bullar boundaries
- After perforating the anteroinferior medial quadrant of the bulla, introduce a small angled curette to seek the boundaries of the bullar cell. Or use a small-jaw 45-degree angled forceps. Use the posterior jaw of the forceps to seek the boundaries before biting.
- The resection of the bone can be performed either with a small angled curette or with angled forceps. Use either instrument to seek the recesses and thin, overlapping bony partitions prior to resection. In this way, step-by-step removal of anterior and medial walls is accomplished.

Surgical significance:
- It is imperative to seek the boundaries of any cell prior to doing any resection. By judging the lateral wall or the lamina papyracea appropriately, one can safely resect the overhanging part of the wall without injuring the lamina papyracea.
- Resection of the bony partitions can be performed either with a small angled curette or with an angled forceps. The Thru-Cut bite forceps work better to prevent mucosal laceration and uneven cuts. Use the posterior or distal part of the jaw of the forceps behind the cell wall, and seek the overhanging part. Hold the biting forceps as if you were seeking or probing the boundaries rather than grabbing.
- Once you feel the recess, assess the overhanging part of the bone and resect with small bites.
- Seeking the boundaries of the bullar cell is very important. It avoids injury to the fovea and ensures resection of the bony partition without causing a crush injury to the neighboring cells. If cells are crushed, they can harbor disease or can cause mucocele formation. Uneven tearing or ripping of the mucosa will induce more bleeding or excessive loss of normal mucosa.

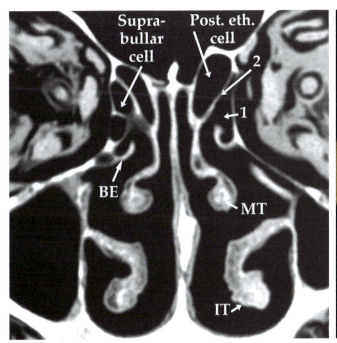
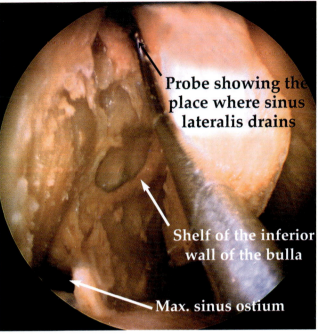

CT section through the midorbital level
1 = Sinus lateralis.
2 = Oblique attachment of the middle turbinate.

In this section, observe the lower shelf of the ethmoid bulla and the number of suprabullar cells. On the right, well-developed suprabullar cells are present. On the left, they are absent. The sinus lateralis is very well developed on the left. Correlate this with the sections on page 7.

Suprabullar cells and the sinus lateralis
- A curved ball probe is used to seek the sinus lateralis. This method seeks the horizontal, oblique, and vertical segments of the basal lamella of the middle turbinate. Careful maneuvering will identify the suprabullar cells. If the suprabullar cells are followed superiorly, one can safely reach the fovea.
- A small shelf of the inferior wall of the bulla is preserved as a landmark to identify the oblique part of the basal lamella. The site of perforation to enter the posterior ethmoid is immediately above and posterior to this shelf.

Surgical significance:
- While exploring the suprabullar cells and the sinus lateralis, one should pull back the endoscope far enough to visualize the maxillary sinus ostium and inferior border of the middle turbinate to obtain a complete overall view. The endoscope should be kept parallel to the inferior border of the middle turbinate. If the endoscope is too close, one can lose the overall view, and foveal injury can occur.
- The maxillary sinus ostium is reconstructed prior to resection of the ethmoid bulla. The reasons for this are:
  1. The anteroinferior surface of the bulla ethmoidalis and the inferior third of the uncinate process serve as landmarks to locate the maxillary sinus ostium.
  2. By following these landmarks (rather than blindly probing) to locate the maxillary sinus ostium, one reduces the incidence of injury to the lamina papyracea. (Now the maxillary sinus ostium serves as a landmark.)
  3. Good depth perception is achieved if the maxillary sinus ostium is kept in view at all times.
  4. The maxillary sinus ostium helps in locating the horizontal attachment of the middle turbinate.

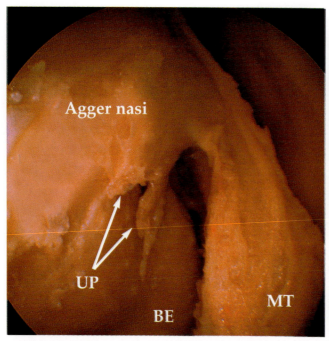
Agger nasi cell

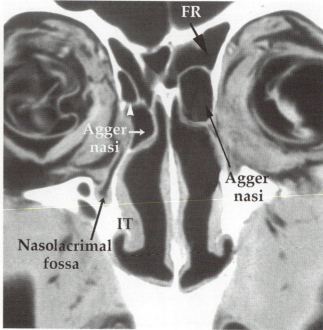
CT section 1 cm posterior to the nasion

After completing the maxillary sinus ostium reconstruction, return to the area of the agger nasi for identification of the upper part of the uncinate process. Next, identify the agger nasi cell. The CT section taken just anterior to the middle turbinate shows agger nasi cells. A true sagittal CT section is difficult to obtain because it requires awkward positioning of the patient. We perform sagittal reconstruction from the coronal acquisition. To obtain reasonably good images, we take 1.5-mm sections at 1.5-mm spacing. The sagittal reconstruction helps us to understand the complex anatomy of the frontal recess.

True sagittal view

Reconstructed sagittal view

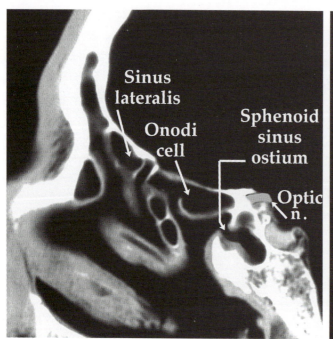
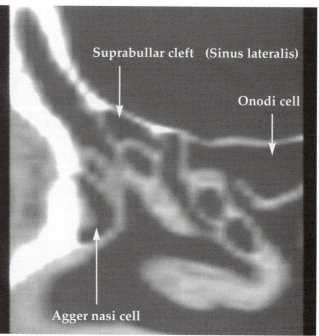

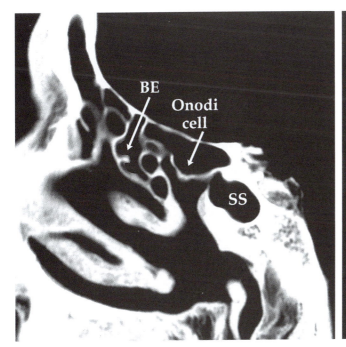 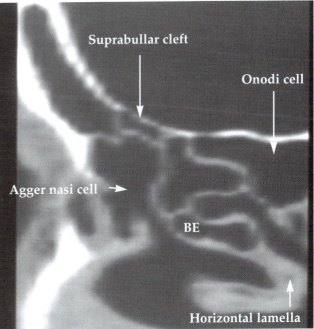

True sagittal CT section
Observe the relationship of the sinus lateralis, the frontal recess, and the agger nasi cell. Note the large posterior ethmoid cell. Posteriorly this cell extends over the sphenoid sinus and comes close to the optic nerve. The cells seen in the basal lamella of the middle turbinate are posterior ethmoid cells. Here, we are able to visualize the sphenoid sinus ostium, which generally is not seen on a CT scan.

Reconstructed sagittal view
- Identify the septate bulla ethmoidalis. The Onodi cell remains superior and lateral to the sphenoid sinus.
- This view depicts the importance of preserving a shelf of the inferior bullar wall. Staying just above the shelf to perforate the oblique part of the basal lamella serves two purposes:
  1. It preserves the integrity of the horizontal attachment of the middle turbinate.
  2. It avoids injury to the fovea.

Surgical significance:
- During the resection of the agger nasi cells, blind grasping with angled forceps should be avoided to prevent injury to the surrounding vital structures. Hence, use the curette to locate the lateral wall and roof of the agger nasi cell, then resect them in an anterior and medial direction.
- Crushing the tissues in the region of the posterosuperior wall of the agger cells will cause subsequent scarring and stenosis in the region of the frontal recess.

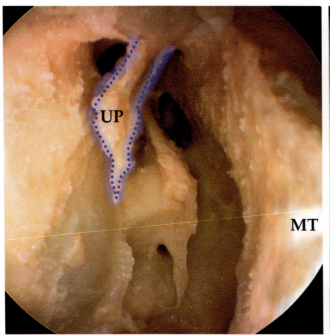

Definition of the upper attachment of the uncinate process

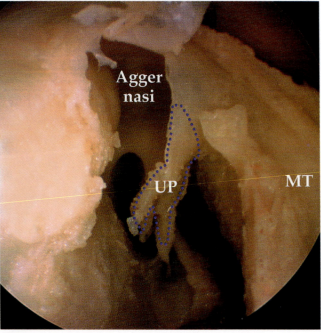

Resected anterior wall of the agger nasi cell

RESECTION OF THE AGGER NASI CELL AND EXPOSURE OF THE FRONTAL RECESS

Resection of the anterior wall of the agger cell is complete. The posterosuperior wall is identified.

Medial part of the posterosuperior wall is resected, exposing the frontal recess and ostium of the midchamber. The remaining wall is removed in the next image.

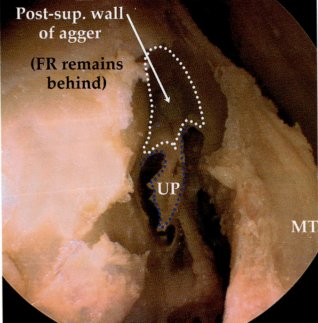

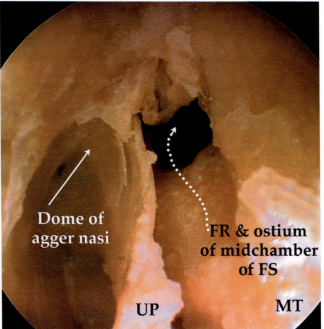

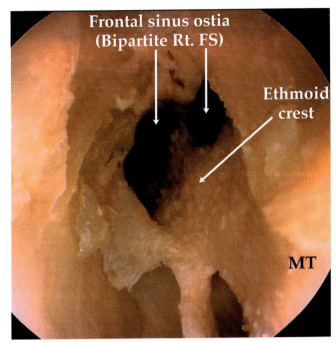
View through a 70-degree endoscope

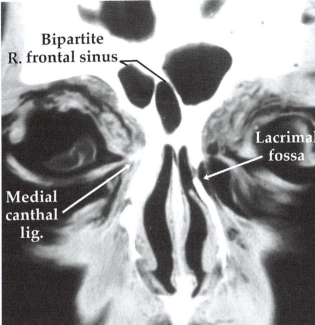
CT section at nasion

- The agger nasi cells are resected next. For this, a small angled curette is used.
- The upper attachments of the uncinate process are identified, and the anterior wall of the agger cell (formed by the lateral merge of the uncinate process) is resected. The anterior wall resection will lead the surgeon to the inside of the agger nasi cell.
- The roof of the agger nasi cell is seen. The remaining anterior part of the uncinate process attachment close to the middle turbinate is resected.
- Next, the posterosuperior wall of the agger cell is identified. This is the wall that is the boundary of the frontal recess.
- The frontal recess is located behind the posterosuperior wall of the agger nasi cells. A portion of this wall is now removed and the frontal sinus ostium is visualized. This ostium represents the midchamber of the frontal sinus. The remaining portion of the wall is resected, exposing the frontal recess and frontal sinus ostium of the right side.
- This resection is possible only in some cases—where the thin, bony partitions are easy to resect with a curette. However, more than 50% of patients will require removal of the bony anterior lateral wall. This is thick bone formed by the ascending process of the maxilla, and its removal requires the use of a diamond bur.

Surgical significance:
- Identification and proper resection of diseased agger nasi cells is imperative to avoid persistent and recurrent disease. CT is the most valuable adjunct for such identification.
- Carefully preserve a small upper part of the uncinate process for identification of the agger nasi area. Sharply resect the mucosa and bony attachment here. This avoids tearing the mucosa and crushing the thin bone, which can obscure the landmark.
- The vertical lamella of the middle turbinate attaches to the lamina cribrosa. This area has the least resistance, particularly when the lateral lamella of the lamina cribrosa is high and thin. Medial maneuvering or dissection should be avoided to prevent injury to the cribriform plate. As a rule, stay strictly lateral to the middle turbinate.
- The lateral wall of the agger cell is the medial wall of the orbit. The resection should therefore be carefully done and limited to the level of the anterior overhang.
- At the same level as above, care should also be taken to avoid injury to the lacrimal sac.

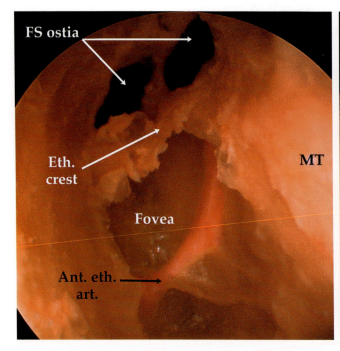
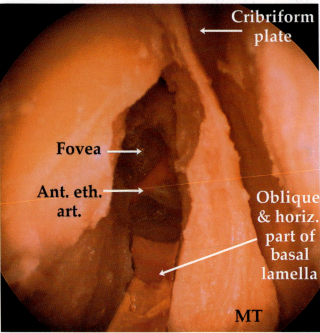

View through a 70-degree endoscope
This shows a clear course of the anterior ethmoid artery, which remains high in the roof with a small bony canal covering it. It enters the roof of the ethmoid laterally from the orbit and then travels anteromedially. It comes close to the ethmoid crest in its most anteromedial portion, where it divides into several branches. The anterior ethmoid fovea is divided by the anterior ethmoid artery into two parts. The anterior part is between the ethmoid crest and the anterior ethmoid artery. The posterior part is posterior to the anterior ethmoid artery.

View through a 0-degree endoscope
- This picture clearly shows the relationship of the upper third of the middle turbinate and the cribriform plate. Correlate this picture with the CT sections on pages 9 and 10. Note the attachment of the vertical part of the middle turbinate to the cribriform plate.
- Vertical, oblique, and horizontal parts of the basal lamella of the middle turbinate are well visualized.

Surgical significance:
- The general belief is that by staying anterior to the anterior ethmoid artery, the surgeon can avoid injury to the brain. This is erroneous. Damage to the anterior fovea can result in such an injury.
- The anterior ethmoid artery sometimes runs with a small mesentery and hangs from the roof. Injury to this part can result in massive hemorrhage and/or cause orbital complications by retraction of the bleeding artery in the orbit.
- The vertical lamella of the middle turbinate is quite often connected to the cribriform plate. Injury at this point leads to CSF rhinorrhea.

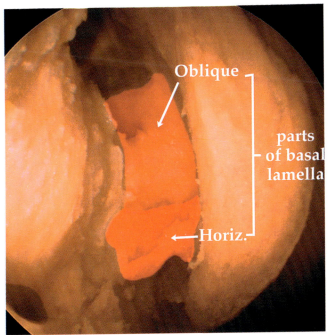
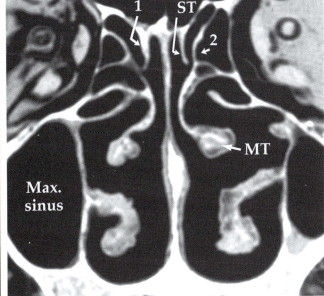

Endoscopic view of the basal lamella
- This section shows two parts of the basal lamella: horizontal and oblique.
- First identify the horizontal part, keeping the endoscope far enough away to visualize the maxillary sinus ostium and the free inferior border of the middle turbinate.
- Identify the junction of the inferior border of the middle turbinate and the lateral wall.
- The entire bony lateral attachment of the horizontal part of the middle turbinate is 1 to 1.5 cm above this point.

CT section through the posterior ethmoid
A coronal CT section shows the oblique attachment of the middle turbinate:
 1 = Superior turbinate.
 2 = Posterior ethmoid cell.

Surgical significance:
- In this section we can identify the oblique and horizontal parts of the basal lamella. It is quite common to injure the horizontal part during identification of the posterior ethmoid cells. Injury to the horizontal part of the basal lamella results in two complications:
  1. Instability of the middle turbinate. This leads to inconvenience during surgery by the flip-flopping middle turbinate, occasional loss of the middle turbinate, and/or postoperative adhesions over the lateral wall.
  2. Hemorrhage as a result of injury to the sphenopalatine artery.
- To identify the oblique part:
  1. Remove the anterior ethmoid cells attached to and obscuring the oblique part.
  2. Using a small curved curette, feel the horizontal part, feel the recesses of the cells, and resect the cells with an anteroinferior motion. Alternatively, a small angled biting forceps may be used to take small bites.
- The oblique part is now well visualized.

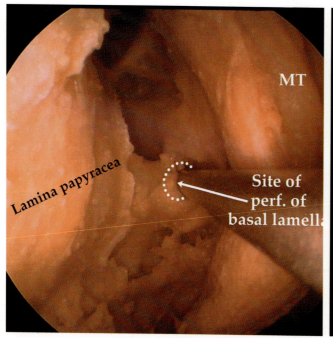 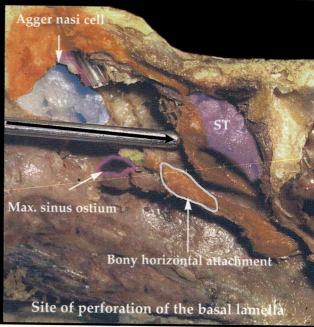

Approach to the posterior ethmoid cells
- This section shows the site of perforation of the oblique part of the basal lamella of the middle turbinate.
- Identify the horizontal attachment.
- Follow it superiorly for a distance of 1 to 1.5 cm.
- Feel the firm bony horizontal attachment of the middle turbinate.
- Direct the perforating instrument almost parallel to the horizontal attachment but not quite (approximately 15 degrees from it). It should point just above the superior edge of the horizontal attachment.
- Perforate close to the turbinate in a medial direction.
- Keep the endoscope parallel to the inferior border of the middle turbinate. Visualize the maxillary sinus ostium.
- After identifying the horizontal and oblique attachments, use a No. 7 Frazier suction or a small straight biting forceps to perforate the oblique part of the basal lamella.
- The perforation site should always be toward the turbinate medially and just superior to the attachment of the horizontal part.

Surgical significance:
- While identifying the basal lamella it is important to keep the endoscope far enough from it to identify the maxillary sinus ostium.
- It is important to identify the horizontal part of the basal lamella because if this part is injured while you are entering the posterior ethmoid cell, you can lose the stability of the middle turbinate. Once the stability of the middle turbinate is lost, it is more likely to lateralize and cause lateral wall adhesions and subsequent recurrence of the disease.
- All the cell partitions should be resected carefully to expose the oblique part of the basal lamella. This is achieved with the use of a curette or a small biting forceps.
- The firm lateral attachment of the basal lamella should be kept intact. Just superior to it at the junction of the oblique with the horizontal part one can perforate the basal lamella to enter into the posterior ethmoid cells.
- The second problem that can occur while perforating the basal lamella is injury to the orbit and the fovea. To avoid this, one should keep the landmarks in view at all times.

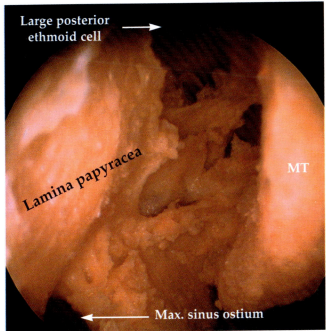
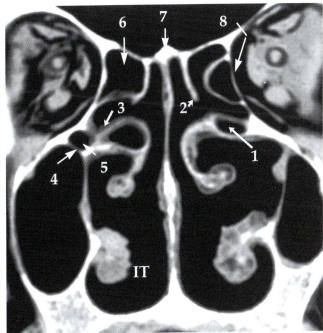

Endoscopic view of the posterior ethmoid
- Once the perforation is made in the basal lamella, insert the angled curette through the perforation and feel the recesses behind the basal lamella to get an idea of the posterior ethmoid cell limits.
- Determine the overhanging portion of the bony partition and then remove it with gentle strokes of the curette in the anteroinferior direction or by taking small bites with the forceps.
- The curette should never be engaged deep behind the cell wall in the lateral or superior direction.

CT section through the horizontal lamella
The section shows:
   1 = Posterior conchal cell.
   2 = Superior turbinate.
   3 = Horizontal attachment of the middle turbinate.
   4 = Ethmoidomaxillary plate.
   5 = Posterior ethmoid cell.
   6 = Fovea ethmoidalis.
   7 = Planum sphenoidale.
   8 = Lamina papyracea.

Surgical significance:
- Identification of the posterior conchal cell is very important. If left behind, the cell can lead to recurring maxillary sinusitis.
- Unroofing this cell by resecting the superior wall can be accomplished with the angled curette turned upside down and entering and perforating the superior wall of this cell.
- The lamina papyracea (lateral wall) should be felt and palpated, then the superior wall. It is useful to develop a tactile sensation for the thin bony plate of the lamina papyracea and the fovea.
- Remove part of the oblique lamella laterally until it merges with the lamina papyracea and superiorly until the fovea is well demonstrated. These areas, if not properly cleaned and clearly visualized, will harbor residual disease.

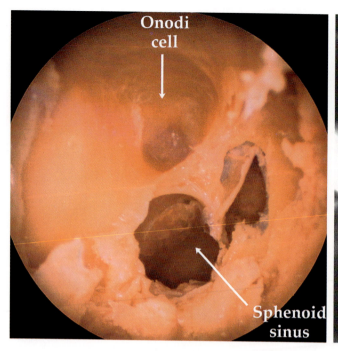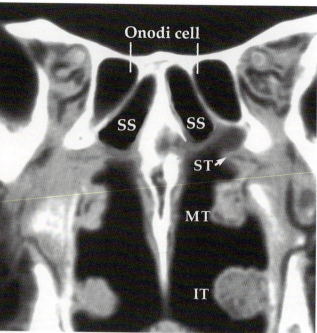

When the oblique lamella is followed superiorly, look for the fovea and the junction of the fovea with the lamina papyracea. The posterior ethmoid artery remains posterior to the junction. The posterior ethmoid artery is not well seen in most cases. The unroofing of the ethmoid cells should be done on the basis of the CT section. Here we see a large Onodi cell that is the posterior ethmoid cell. It extends posterosuperiorly over the sphenoid sinus. The optic nerve usually lies in the wall of the Onodi cell when it is present, and hence is more liable to injury when dissection is done from anterior to posterior—i.e., when an attempt is made to enter the sphenoid through the posterior ethmoid cells. To avoid any injury to the optic nerve, one should carefully study the CT section and identify the Onodi cell and posterior ethmoid cell extension. After removing the diseased tissue, enter the sphenoid sinus by coming forward into the anteroinferior medial segment. Using a small angled curette, perforate the sphenoid sinus. This is the transethmoid approach to the sphenoid sinus. Partly resect the partition wall between the sphenoid sinus and posterior ethmoid cell (Onodi cell). Both cavities are now connected.

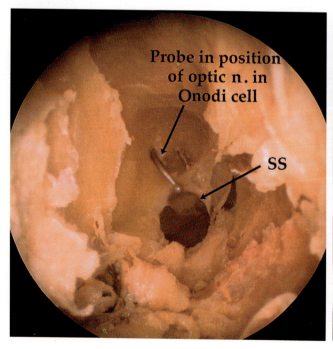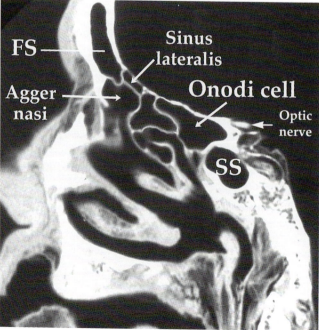

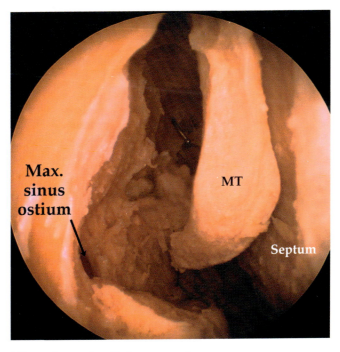

View through a 0-degree endoscope

This should be the final view after total ethmoidectomy with maxillary sinusotomy and sphenoidotomy. One should be able to see the entire ethmoid cavity from the anterior to the posterior segment without any obstruction. Also, one should be able to see the reconstructed maxillary sinus ostium.

Surgical significance:
- The middle turbinate should remain stable and should not flop up toward the lateral wall. This indicates stability of its vertical and horizontal attachments.
- The photo also shows a probe that was placed at the course of the optic nerve through the Onodi cell wall. It is at the junction of the lateral and the posterior walls.
- The cavity is covered with a water-soluble antibiotic ointment such as Bactroban or Betadine.
- If the stability of the middle turbinate is quite good, spacers may not be needed.
- This concludes the surgery.
- Postoperatively, periodically debride the cavity with the help of a 0- or 30-degree endoscope, No. 7 Frazier suction, and small biting forceps until the healing is complete.

2
CORONAL-SECTIONAL ANATOMY WITH CT SECTION CORRELATIONS

This chapter will present and discuss various coronal CT sections that are indispensable in sinus surgery. It also will correlate these sections with actual cadaveric anatomy.

We use a General Electric Hi-Light Advantage CT scan unit at Sherman Hospital. Axial or coronal images of the sinuses are obtained using 1.5-mm collimation and 4.0-mm spacing. Detail scan technique is utilized and the display field of view is generally 16 cm for adults and 14 cm for children. In the axial plane, scans are obtained from the inferior aspect of the maxillary sinuses (usually slightly below the level of the hard palate) through the top of the frontal sinuses. In the coronal plane (perpendicular to the hard palate is optimal), scans are obtained from the nasion to the posterior aspect of the sphenoid sinus. Intravenous contrast is not normally used for CT evaluation of a routine case of rhinosinusitis. However, if the patient has a history of, or is strongly suspected of having, pyocele, mucocele or paranasal sinus malignancy, then intravenous contrast is essential.

Filming of the CT images is best done with a modified bone window. We use a window width of 4000 H.U. and a window level of 150 H.U. This setting is best for visualizing mucosal pathology of the paranasal sinuses. However, this setting is not optimal for evaluation of surrounding soft tissues of the face and orbits. One can supplement the modified bone windows with soft tissue windows (window width 500, window level 85) if desired. If intravenous contrast is used (see above) then supplemental soft tissue windows are mandatory.

We have several different scan protocols. A full sinus CT scan would entail both axial and coronal scans (1.5-mm thick with 4.0-mm spacing). Our screening study is coronal images only (1.5-mm thick with 8.0-mm spacing). Finally, we have a study that is well suited as a pre-endoscopic nasal surgery study. We call this our "ethmoid series" and it consists of coronal images of 1.5-mm-thick slices with 4.0-mm spacing. If the patient has had prior surgery or if disease of the frontal or sphenoid sinus is suspected, then a full sinus CT scan should be performed. If intravenous contrast is used (see above), a full sinus CT scan should be performed.

It is sometimes helpful to have sagittal reconstructions made of the paranasal sinuses. The sagittal images can be helpful in demonstrating the relationship of the agger nasi cells to the frontal recess. Sagittal reconstructions are best if they are made from the coronal acquisition. The coronal images should be acquired at 1.5-mm collimation and at 1.5-mm spacing. Direct sagittal images of the sinuses are technically difficult to acquire.

Anterior view of the section

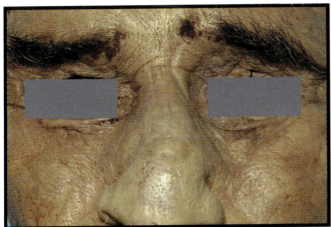

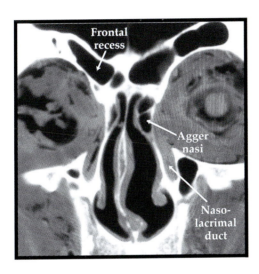

Posterior view of the section

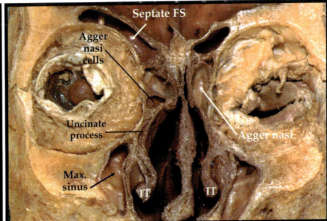

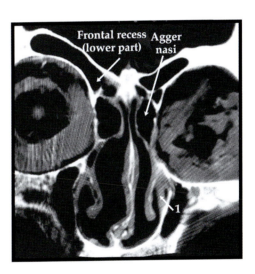

The section at the level of the nasion is very important. In this section, study the frontal recess and the arrangement of the agger nasi cells. The lacrimal sac and part of the nasolacrimal duct are shown. The size of the agger cells determines the amount of working space for the exploration of the frontal recess. Do not overlook the position of the nasal septum. The surgical approach to the agger cells, the frontal recess, and the lacrimal sac is cumbersome and difficult in the presence of an upper deviation of the septum.

This section is 1 cm posterior to the nasion. It is also anterior to the anterior surface of the middle turbinate. The uncinate process merges anteriorly with the lateral nasal wall. Superiorly it continues into the medial wall of the agger nasi cells and attaches to the middle turbinate, the lamina papyracea, and the fovea. Look for the frontal recess and its relationship to the agger cells.

Anterior view of the section   **Posterior view of the section**

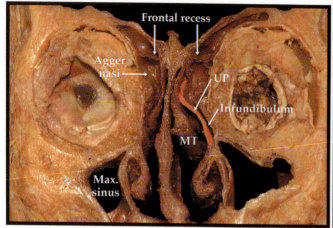

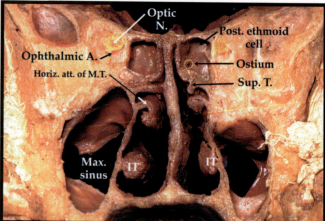

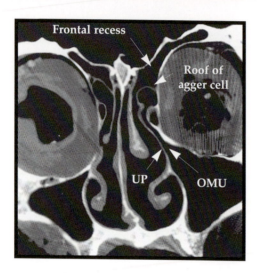

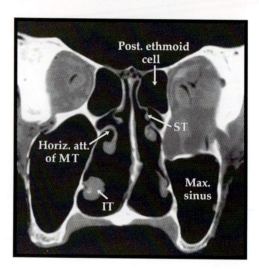

The above section shows the relations of the uncinate process. Superiorly it merges with the dome of the agger cells. It attaches medially to the middle turbinate and laterally to the lamina papyracea. The inferior third of the uncinate process is of critical importance. In over 90% of cases, the natural ostium of the maxillary sinus is located posterior to it. Note the difference in height between the cribriform plate and the fovea. The depth of the olfactory fossa varies considerably from person to person and from side to side, and the olfactory fossa is at a much lower level than the ethmoid fovea. The vertical lamella of the middle turbinate attaches to the cribriform plate.

This section is through the posterior ethmoid sinus just posterior to the oblique part of the basal lamella of the middle turbinate. Here, it is made up of one large posterior cell. At this level, the optic nerve remains apart from the lateral wall of the posterior ethmoid cell. However, as we go posterior, it gets closer. This can be seen in later sections. The horizontal part of the basal lamella of the middle turbinate is clearly seen here. Asymmetrical maxillary sinuses, as seen here, are not unusual.

Anterior view of the section	Posterior view of the section
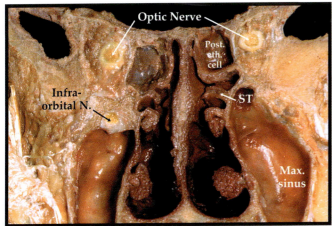	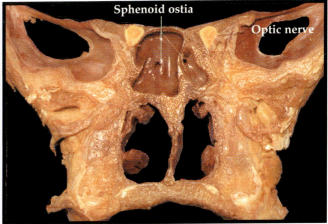
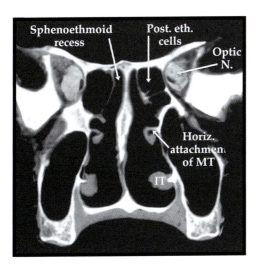	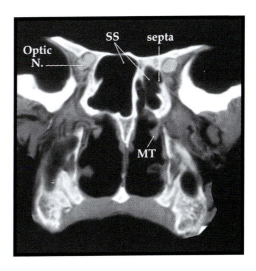

In this section we see the posterior ethmoid cells and their relationship to the optic nerve. It is of utmost importance to ensure that the bony partition between these two structures remains intact. Identify the horizontal attachment of the middle turbinate and the superior turbinate. The most posterior and superior recess in the nasal cavity is the sphenoethmoid recess. The sphenoid sinus and cells of the posterior ethmoid sinus drain into this recess. Study this area very carefully.

Study of this section is necessary to determine the integrity of the lateral and superior walls of the sphenoid sinus, especially in relation to the optic nerve. Injury to this area can result in blindness. The septum of the sphenoid sinus is rarely in the midline, which results in asymmetrical sinuses. Occasionally on its posterior side, the septum attaches to the carotid canal. Injury to this area can result in death. In coronal views one cannot see the ostium of the sphenoid sinus. For a more detailed sphenoid study, an axial scan should be included with a 4-mm spacing from the frontal sinus to the hard palate.

Anterior view of the section   **Posterior view of the section**

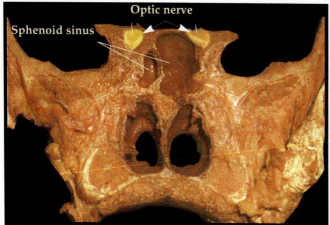
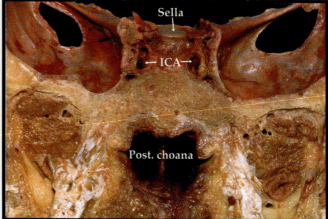

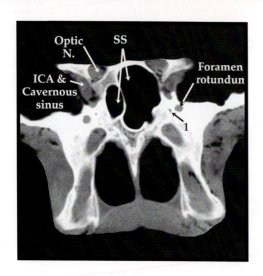
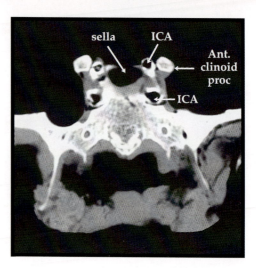

This section shows the relationship of the sphenoid sinus to the internal carotid artery and the optic nerve. Also of interest is the foramen rotundum, through which passes the maxillary division of the trigeminal nerve.
The above CT section shows:
    1 = Pterygopalatine foramen, through which the vidian nerve passes.
    2 = Medial and lateral pterygoid plates.
    3 = Rostrum of the sphenoid.

This section is posterior to the sphenoid sinus. Note the location of the sella turcica and the internal carotid artery. Note also the anterior clinoid process.

Anterior view of the section

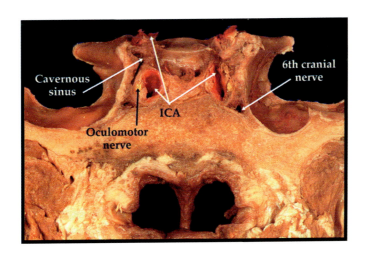

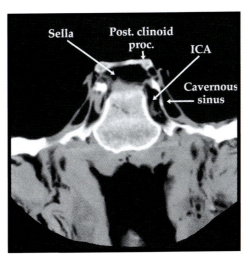

This is the posteriormost section through the nasopharynx. Part of the sella turcica, the posterior clinoid process, and the serpentine course of the internal carotid artery can be clearly seen. The cavernous sinus is located close to the sphenoid sinus and the sella turcica. Its contents from the superior to the inferior direction are the internal carotid artery and cranial nerves III (the oculomotor nerve), IV (the trochlear nerve), the ophthalmic division of V (the trigeminal nerve), and VI (the abducens nerve).

3
REGIONAL SURGICAL ANATOMY

The lateral nasal wall is formed by the ethmoid, the maxilla, the palatine, the lacrimal, the medial pterygoid plate of the sphenoid, the nasal and the inferior turbinate bones. The middle, superior, and, when present, the supreme turbinates are projections of the ethmoid bone that further contribute to the formation of the lateral nasal wall. Each turbinate overlies a small air space beneath its attachment and lateral to it known as the meatus.

ETHMOID SINUS

An integral part of the ethmoid sinus is formed by bony lamellae. These form partitions which:
- Separate cells into different groups.
- Provide attachments to the turbinates. There are four turbinates: inferior, middle, superior and supreme. There are two secondary turbinates, the ethmoid bulla and the uncinate process.

The inferior turbinate is the largest. The middle turbinate is the most central. Its ground plate divides the ethmoid into two sections: anterior cells, which drain into the middle meatus, and posterior cells, which drain into the superior meatus. These groups of cells tend to invade each other's zone by pushing aside the lamellar barrier. The integrity of the barrier, though, is always maintained, so the cells do not communicate, and they maintain their own drainage system. Anatomical variations in the form of unusual cell extensions are quite common.

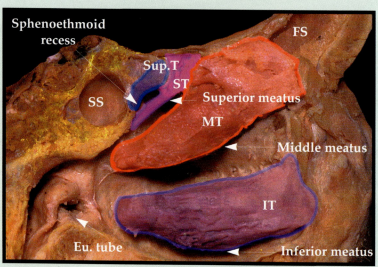

These cells have a great tendency to infringe upon adjacent structures. This infringement may be:
I. Intramural
   A. Invasion of the bulla by the anterior group of cells.
   B. Invasion of the posterior area by the bullar cells, causing flattening of the posterior cells. This occurs in 10% of cases.
II. Extramural
   Ethmoid cells can grow in any and all directions until they encounter hard bone. They may:
   A. Pneumatize the supraorbital plate of the frontal bone, producing a supraorbital cell (15%).
   B. Encroach on the floor of the frontal sinus, producing a bulge known as a "frontal bulla."
   C. Encroach on the crista galli and uncinate process occasionally.
   D. Extend into the middle turbinate, producing a concha bullosa and nasal septum, and may pass through the nasal septum to the other side.
   E. Invade the infraorbital plate of the maxilla, producing an infraorbital ethmoid cell (Haller's cells, 10%).
   F. Extend posterosuperiorly to the sphenoid sinus, known as sphenoethmoid cell (Onodi cell, 10%).

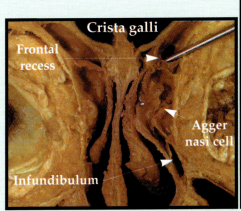 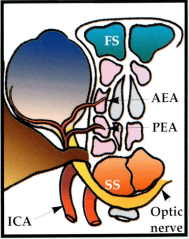 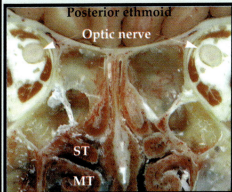

CHARACTERISTICS OF THE ETHMOID SINUS

Development: Develops from several mucosal projections from the fetal nasal chamber. Development begins at about the fifth fetal month. By the seventh month, the different ethmoid groups are recognizable.
In the newborn the cells are round. By the second year, they have elongated toward the frontal bone. By the seventh year, the cells have gradually enlarged, reducing the intracellular septa to thin, fragile laminae of compact bone.
By the thirteenth or fourteenth year, the ethmoid has reached the limit of expansion.

Pneumatization & Growth: Pneumatization starts in the vertical segment and continues for one to twenty years.

Properties:
- The ethmoid sinus is pyramidal in shape with a honeycomb appearance. It fits between the lacrimal bone anteriorly and the sphenoid bone posteriorly.
- It is structurally intricate and extremely variable, often asymmetrical.
- The roof slants downward posteroanteriorly at an angle of 15 degrees.
- The anterior two-thirds is constituted by frontal bone, foveolae ethmoidalis, which is thick and dense.
- The roof curves downward to join the cribriform plate. This junction is one-tenth as strong as the roof (Stammberger). The roof is higher laterally than medially. The highest point of the roof is higher than the cribriform plate by as much as 15-17 mm.
- The cribriform plate is very thin and is perforated in many places by the filia olfactoria.
- Some natural dehiscences are seen, both in the anterior ethmoid canal and in the roof of the ethmoid (tertiary canals).

Adult Size (Average): 3.3 x 2.7 x 1.4 cm.

Surgical significance: The size and shape of the sinus vary considerably. Hence it is important to study the CT scan to delineate the sinus. One should remember that the posteriorly sloping roof of the sinus may not be symmetrical on both sides, and its medial junction with the thin cribriform plate presents a risk of penetration at surgery. To avoid injury one should clearly define the lamina of the middle turbinate and stay lateral to it. Natural dehiscences may be present in the lamina papyracea. The invading properties of the ethmoid cells make it difficult to identify the basal lamella of the middle turbinate. Extreme care is needed during surgery because there is very little distance between the posterior wall of the invading bullar cell and the sphenoid sinus. Similar difficulties are encountered when the posterior cells invade the bullar cells.

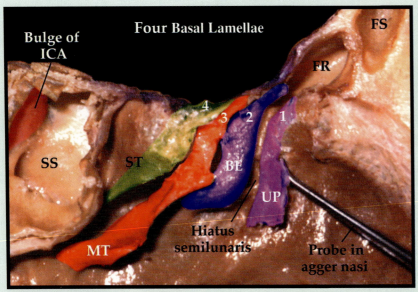

Basal Lamella (Ground Lamella)
During endoscopic sinus surgery a sequence of bony landmarks is encountered. These are:
1. Uncinate process.
2. Bulla ethmoidalis.
3. Basal lamella of the middle turbinate.
4. Lamella of the superior turbinate.
5. Lamella of the supreme turbinate when present. Nos. 1 and 2 are considered secondary turbinates.

Anatomically and physiologically the middle turbinate is considered to be the most important of the basal lamellae. It divides the ethmoid into anterior and posterior complexes.

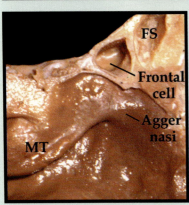

Uncinate Process
The uncinate process is a sickle-shaped, thin, bony plate that runs in an anterosuperior to posteroinferior direction. It looks like a slightly bent hook.
Attachments:
    Anterior: Anterosuperiorly it attaches to the middle turbinate, thus forming the inferomedial wall of the agger cell.
    Inferior: Inferior turbinate and the palatine bone.
    Posterior: Free margin is concave and runs parallel to the curvature of the bulla ethmoidalis.
    Superior: May attach to the lacrimal bone. The uppermost portion may be attached to the base of the skull or the lamina papyracea. It almost always fuses with the middle turbinate anterosuperiorly.

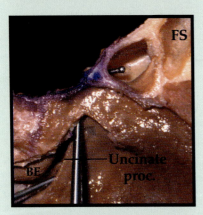

Hiatus Semilunaris Inferior (Zuckerkandl)
- Sickle-shaped two-dimensional cleft.
- The average width is 1.5 mm. It is bounded by the concave, free posterior margin of the uncinate process and the anterior surface of the bulla ethmoidalis.
- The lateral wall is made up of the lamina papyracea, particularly in the inferior half. Anterosuperiorly it may end in the frontal recess.
- Anteroinferiorly it may end in a three-dimensional space where the maxillary sinus ostium is located. This space is known as the ethmoid infundibulum.

Hiatus Semilunaris Superior
- The space between the bulla ethmoidalis and the middle turbinate.
- The suprabullar recess, when present, opens into it.

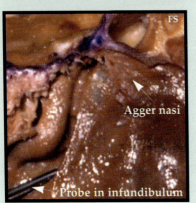

Ethmoid Infundibulum
A space, which may be a well-defined three-dimensional cleft, located in the anteroinferior segment of the hiatus semilunaris.
The natural ostium of the maxillary sinus opens into this space.
    Medial wall—uncinate process.
    Lateral wall—formed by the lamina papyracea, the frontal process of the maxilla and occasionally by the lacrimal bone.
    Depth—the average depth is 2 mm. It varies from 0.5 to 10 mm. It is measured at the site of the maxillary ostium and depends on the size and height of the uncinate process.

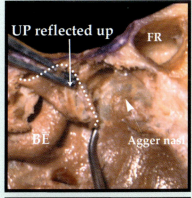

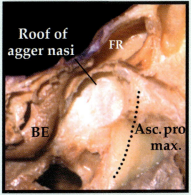

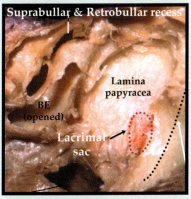

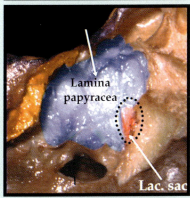

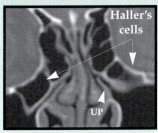

Agger Nasi Cell
- Smooth elevation anterior and superior to the junction of the middle turbinate with the lateral nasal wall. A remnant of the first ethmoturbinal.
- Product of pneumatization of the lacrimal bone, which forms its lateral surface. Most frequently pneumatized cell.
- The first cell to pneumatize in the newborn, it remains very prominent in children.
- 1 to 3 cells.
- The uncinate process merges anterosuperiorly into the lateral nasal wall, hiding the agger nasi cell.
- The cell occasionally extends into the ascending process of the maxilla and the floor of the frontal sinus and, rarely, into the nasal bone.
- The posterosuperior wall of the cell forms the inferior wall of the frontal recess. Refer to page 45.

Ethmoid Bulla
- The most constant landmark.
- Generally the largest air cell in the anterior ethmoid. Rarely absent.
- Minimal or no pneumatization in 8% of cases (Stammberger). A bony ridge or bulge, the torus lateralis, occurs in 40% of cases (Zuckerkandl and Grünwald).
- Boundaries:

  Anterior: Convex curvature is parallel to the posterior free border of the uncinate process.
  Superior: Fovea. Either by a single cell or by one or two suprabullar cells. Anterior bullar wall forms the posterior wall of the frontal recess. Suprabullar space (sinus lateralis). When this space is well formed, the frontal sinus drains into it.
  Posterior: Basal lamella, for a varied distance.
  Lateral: Lamina papyracea.
  Medial: Covered by the middle turbinate.

Suprabullar and Retrobullar Recess (Sinus Lateralis—Grünwald)
- Cleft between the roof of the ethmoid, ground lamella and the bulla.
- Not always present.
- When well pneumatized, the ethmoid bulla opens into it.
- Boundaries:

  Superior: Fovea.
  Inferior: Roof of the ethmoid bulla.
  Posterior: Basal lamella of the middle turbinate.
  Lateral: Lamina papyracea.
  Medial: Middle turbinate.
  Dorsal: Space between the bulla ethmoidalis and the basal lamella.
  Opens: Between bulla ethmoidalis and middle turbinate, in a space known as the "hiatus semilunaris superior" ("recess suprabullaris"—Hajek).

Infraorbital Ethmoid Cell (Haller's Cell)
- Pneumatized cells present in the roof of the maxillary sinus (orbital floor).
- Generally localized in the anterior ethmoid. May extend all the way from the anterior to the posterior ethmoid.
- Distinct from the bulla and the maxillary sinus.
- Can cause narrowing of the infundibulum. Refer to page 41.

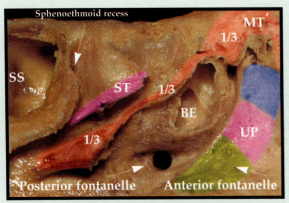 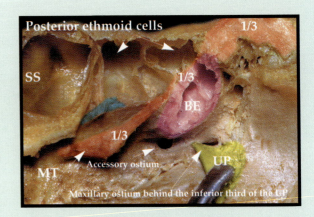

Basal Lamella of the Middle Turbinate.
- Originates from the third basal lamella of the ethmoturbinals.
- Three parts:

Three parts:	Plane	Attachments
Anterior one-third	Vertical (sagittal plane)	Crista ethmoidalis and the skull base
Middle one-third	Oblique (frontal plane)	Lamina papyracea
Posterior one-third	Horizontal (horizontal plane)	Lamina papyracea & lamina perpendicularis

- It divides the ethmoid complex into anterior and posterior groups. Its position varies depending on the pneumatization of the anterior and posterior ethmoid. The anterior ethmoid group opens into the middle meatus. The posterior ethmoid group opens into the superior meatus.
- *Surgical significance:* One should enter the posterior ethmoid through the oblique part close to its junction with the horizontal part. Injury to the other two parts destabilizes the middle turbinate.

Nasal Fontanelles
- Two distinct areas on the lateral nasal wall where the nasal mucosa and the mucoperiosteum of the maxillary sinus are in intimate contact without the presence of any bone.
- The anterior fontanelle is anterior and inferior to the inferior attachment of the uncinate process.
- The posterior fontanelle lies superior to the posterior insertion of the uncinate process.

Concha Bullosa
- Pneumatized middle turbinate. Its size varies.
- A normal variant may cause crowding of the middle meatus. This may predispose to obstruction of the ostiomeatal unit.

Interlamellar Cell
- Pneumatized cell in the vertical lamella of the middle turbinate.
- Pneumatization originates from the superior meatus.

Supraorbital Ethmoid Cells
- Extramural invasion of the supraorbital plate of the frontal bone by air cells of the ethmoid sinus (15%-21%).

Posterior Ethmoid
- The size of the posterior ethmoid depends on its encroachment anteriorly by the anterior ethmoid cells and posteriorly by the sphenoid.
- The number of cells varies from 1 to 5. They are larger and fewer in number than the anterior ethmoid cells.

Sphenoethmoid Cell
- Posterosuperior ethmoid cell (also known as Onodi cell) that extends beyond the sphenoid. When present, it has an intimate relationship with the optic nerve and/or internal carotid artery. This is the most common spot of injury to the optic nerve. To avoid injury to the optic nerve, stay medial and inferior after perforation of the basal lamella.

Optic Nerve Tubercle
- Bony protuberance on the medial surface of the optic foramen. The degree of pneumatization varies. It may surround the optic nerve and predispose it to surgical trauma during endoscopic posterior ethmoidectomy.

Ethmoid Roof

- The anterior two-thirds is constituted by the frontal bone, the fovea ethmoidalis, which is thick and dense. Average thickness is 0.5 mm.
- It slants posteriorly at a 15-degree angle.
- Medially it joins the lamina cribrosa, forming a very fragile junction. It is considered to be one-tenth as strong as the roof. To avoid injury one should clearly define the lamina of the middle turbinate and stay lateral to it.
- Laterally it attaches to a thin paperlike bone called the lamina papyracea.
- The height of the roof varies considerably even from one side to the other. It can be as high as 15 to 17 mm above the cribriform plate. The medial slope of the roof also varies on both sides. Therefore, medial manipulation in the ethmoid cavity without identifying the landmarks can cause injury to the cribriform plate and the dura.
- Keros has differentiated the ethmoid roof configuration based on the length of the lateral lamella of the cribriform plate, as shown below.

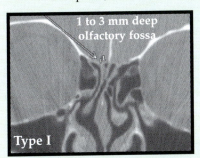 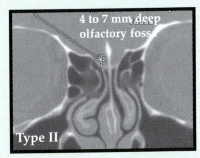 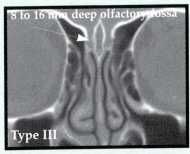

Other variations and asymmetry in the ethmoid roof

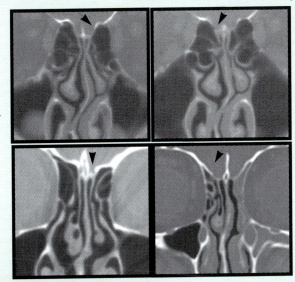 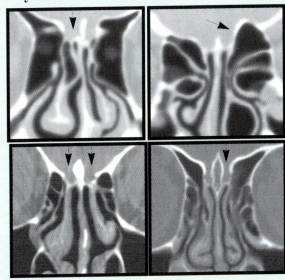

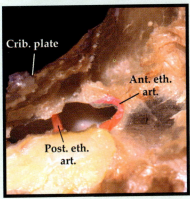

Anterior Ethmoid Artery

- It originates from the ophthalmic artery, enters the anterior ethmoid, and generally remains in the bony canal (ethmoid canal is 4-15 mm), traversing from the lateral side anteromedially into the nose. It then enters medially into the lamina cribrosa. It remains extradural from here to the olfactory fossa. According to Stammberger, bony dehiscences in this area are found in 20% to 40% of cases and the anterior ethmoid artery is a single vessel on both sides in 75% of cases.

Posterior Ethmoid Artery

- After arising from the ophthalmic artery, it enters the posterior ethmoid and travels anteromedially in a bony canal (the posterior ethmoid canal). The distance between this canal and the optic foramen varies from 5 to 10 mm.

Maxillary Sinus

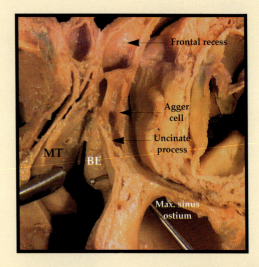 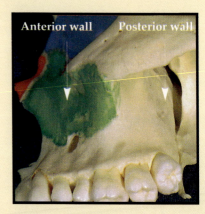 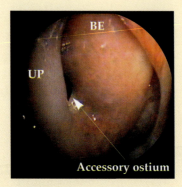

Anterior Wall
- Infraorbital foramen located in its midsuperior part, below the orbital rim. Infraorbital nerve passes through it.
- Inferior margin is indented by teeth. The part above the canine tooth is the thinnest—the canine fossa.

Posterior Wall
- Thicker laterally than medially.
- Behind this wall is the pterygomaxillary fossa and its contents: (1) internal maxillary artery and its branches, (2) sphenopalatine ganglion and the vidian canal, (3) greater palatine nerve, and (4) foramen rotundum.

Roof
- The infraorbital nerve runs through the infraorbital canal in the midsection of the roof. This canal is reported to be dehiscent in 14% of cases.
- It is quite thin on both sides of the infraorbital canal.

Floor
- Composed of the alveolar and palatine processes of the maxilla.
- Level varies with that of the nasal floor. Generally at 9 years of age the sinus floor is at the same level as the nasal floor. Before age 9 the sinus floor is at a higher level. As growth continues, after age 9 the sinus floor is at lower level than the nasal floor.
- The most constant relationship is with the three molar teeth. Closest is the first molar.

Nasolacrimal Duct
- The maxillary ostium is in close proximity to it. On average it lies 4 mm posterior to the duct (1.3-11.5 mm —Lang), average distance 9±3 mm (1.8-18 mm—Calhoun).

Accessory Ostium
- It is a nonfunctional extra opening of the maxillary sinus in the lateral wall of the nose.
- Its number may vary from 1 to 5 and its incidence is 4% to 41%.
- It is usually located in the posterior fontanelle but may be found at other sites such as the anterior fontanelle and the uncinate process.
- It is believed by some authors to result from infections of the maxillary sinus and breakdown of its membranous part. However, I have seen accessory ostia in numerous healthy maxillary sinuses.

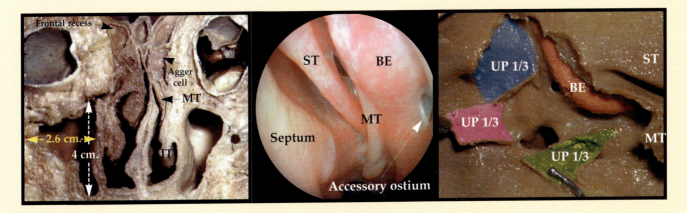

CHARACTERISTICS OF THE MAXILLARY SINUS

Development: Develops from an invagination of the nasal mucous membrane into the maxillary bone. Development begins in third fetal month.

Agenesis: Bilateral—very rare.
Unilateral—occasional.

Pneumatization & Growth: Pneumatization starts at birth. Growth continues up to 18 years of age. Asymmetrical.

Chambers: Usually, one on each side.
Two or more chambers may be present on one or both sides: 1% to 6%.
Asymmetry and unilateral hypoplasia are not uncommon. Complete aplasia is rare.
Thin bony intrasinus septa, complete or incomplete, are not uncommon.

Adult Size (Average):

	Van Alyea	Lang (Right sinus)	Lang (Left sinus)
Height (mm)	33	40.0	40.8
Width (mm)	23	26.2	26.9
Depth (mm) (Anteroposterior)	34	38.4	39.1

Dimensions at various ages (Lang):

Age (year)	1	3	5	8	10	12	14	18
Height (average, in mm)	12.5	18	20.0	24	27	29	30.0	40.4
Width (average, in mm)	12.0	18	20.5	23	27	28	28.5	26.4

Capacity (ml): 14.75 (Schaeffer)

Surgical significance: This sinus, also known as the antrum of Highmore, is the largest of all paranasal sinuses. It is present at birth. The location of its ostium, high in the infundibulum, makes it vulnerable to infections. Its intimate relationship with the molar teeth also makes it more prone to infections.

Maxillary Ostium

- The natural maxillary ostium is located in the ethmoid infundibulum, which is a three-dimensional space in the hiatus semilunaris lateral to the uncinate process. The depth of this space is measured at the site of the maxillary ostium and depends on the size and height of the uncinate process. Its average depth is 2 mm and varies from 0.5 to 10 mm.
- The ostium may be vertically (57.6%), horizontally (20%) or obliquely (3.4%) placed (Mayerson).
- Its average size is 2.4 mm and varies from 1 to 11x17 mm.

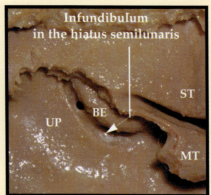

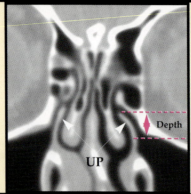

Access to Maxillary Ostium

- Depends on the depth of the infundibulum and whether the ostium is situated vertically, horizontally or obliquely in the infundibulum.
- First define the depth of the hiatus semilunaris with a 70-degree bent ball probe.
- Next, anchor the uncinate process with the probe and define the mobile part of the uncinate process by wiggling it. This is an important step for planning the incision for uncinectomy.
- The lower third of the uncinate process is reflected to reveal the maxillary sinus ostium.

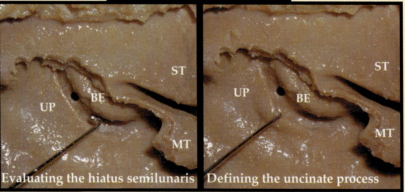

Evaluating the hiatus semilunaris   Defining the uncinate process

- An ostium longer than 3 mm is considered a canal. Its incidence is 83%. It travels posteroinferiorly into the maxillary sinus in 82% of cases and anteroinferiorly in 18%.
- An ostium shorter than 3 mm is referred to as an ostium. Its occurrence is 17% (Simon).

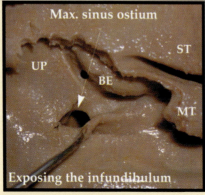

Exposing the infundibulum

A 70-degree bent ball probe seen here is prepared from Allport Mastoid Search 6-1/4" probe (AU5680 Baxter - V. Mueller product). This probe comes with a 90-degree bend. When bent at 70 degrees it becomes an ideal instrument for the infundibulum.

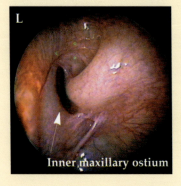

Inner maxillary ostium

The uncinate process has three layers: the inner mucosal layer, the middle bony layer and the outer mucosal layer. The inner mucosal layer is also the medial mucosal wall of the infundibulum. In performing a partial uncinectomy the inner mucosal layer is very carefully preserved and reflected inferiorly over the inferior turbinate.

Endoscopic view of the left inner maxillary ostium. The maxillary ostium is located close to the junction of the roof of the maxilla and lamina papyracea.

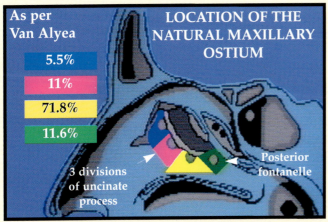

Over 88% of the natural ostium of the maxillary sinus remains hidden behind the uncinate process. Hence, it is not visible through the endoscope.

This diagram depicts the four possible locations of the natural ostium. Professor Van Alyea reported that statistically most ostia are behind the lower one-third of the uncinate process. A similar percentage was reported by Professor Lang more recently.

Based on this anatomical fact, I have designed a technique of "infundibulotomy through Nick's triangle." A precise partial uncinectomy is performed to expose the ethmoid infundibulum. The natural maxillary ostium is identified with the least possible trauma to the inner ostial mucosa. In an inflamed condition, if the ostium is not visible, use the ball probe, passing it along the mucosa of the orbital curvature to locate it. Reconstruction of the ostium is performed based on the amount of pathology.
Partial uncinectomy avoids injury to the frontal recess and preserves mucosa and ethmoid cellular anatomy.

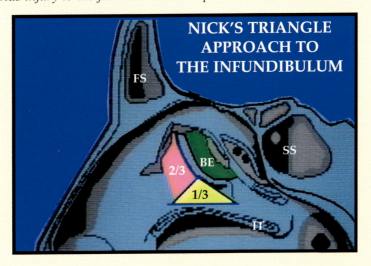

Nick's Triangle

To map out this triangle, first identify and define the uncinate process. Make the first cut above the inferior turbinate and parallel to it through the mucosa down to the bony uncinate plate. The free edge of the uncinate process is the second line of the triangle. To complete the triangle, resect the inferior one-third of the uncinate process layer by layer. This constitutes Nick's triangle. The inner mucosal layer of the uncinate process is very carefully preserved and reflected inferiorly over the inferior turbinate. This step makes the partial uncinectomy a safer procedure because by following the mucosal lining without interrupting or damaging it, it is easier to identify the inner maxillary ostium. It also avoids injury to the orbit.

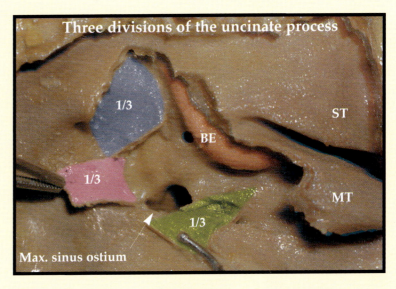

39

Variations of the Infundibular Anatomy on CT Scan

Radiological evaluation of the infundibular space is of utmost importance since the maxillary ostium is located here. Endoscopic access to the ostium varies according to the size and condition of the uncinate plate and whether the ostium is situated obliquely, vertically or horizontally in the infundibulum. The following CT scans demonstrate the variations.

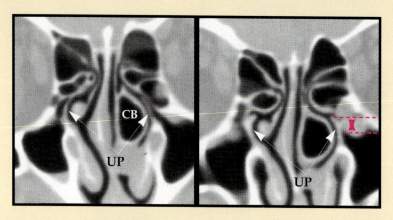

The infundibulum
The wall of the uncinate process is 2 mm high (70% of cases—Van Alyea).

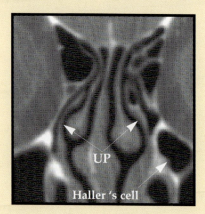

Deep and narrow infundibulum
The wall of the uncinate process is more than 4 mm high (25% of cases—Van Alyea).
The space between the uncinate wall and the lamina papyracea is extremely narrow on the right (7%—Van Alyea) and of average depth on the left side.
The ostium is not seen on this 4-mm sectional study. It appears to be obstructed by the Haller's cell on the left side.

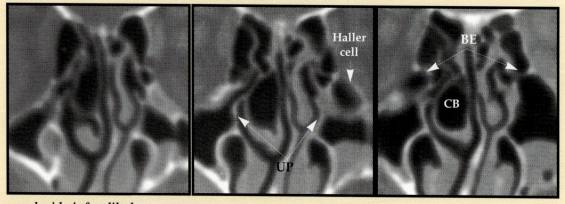

Shallow and wide infundibulum
The wall of the uncinate process is less than 2 mm high (5% of cases—Van Alyea).

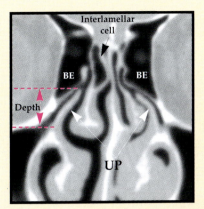
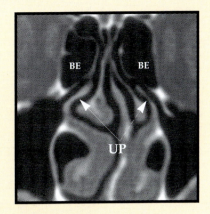

Overhanging bulla with deep and narrow infundibulum
The tall uncinate process hugs the bulla, making the infundibulum a long, narrow channel.

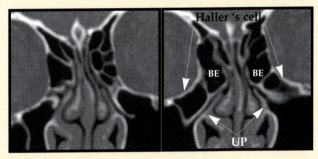

Overhanging Haller's cell with deep and narrow infundibulum
The tall uncinate process hugs the Haller's cell and the bulla, making the infundibulum a long narrow channel.

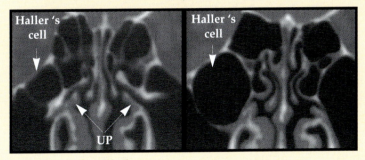

Giant Haller's cell with shallow infundibulum

Surgical significance:
- These anatomical variations seen on the CT scans serve as indicators of the difficulty the surgeon will encounter in locating the ostium. For instance, in a long narrow infundibulum or in the presence of a large Haller's cell, access to the ostium is more difficult, though not impossible.
- In a diseased state with anatomical abnormalities, identification of the ostium becomes difficult. Anatomical knowledge and a careful review of the preoperative CT scan help to define the ostium and its pathology.
- The diseased ostium is obstructed by the inflamed mucoperiosteum. One misstep, either by a sharp instrument or by an overaggressive move, will lacerate the mucosa, cause bleeding and obscure the view. This can then result in a false passage or injury to the orbit.
- The way to avoid these problems is to be very precise in approaching the infundibulum. This precision can be achieved by using the Nick's triangle technique to address the infundibulum. The instrumentation that is ideally suited for this approach is the KTP/532 laser followed by the microdebrider.
- A deep and narrow infundibulum with anatomical variations like the Haller's cell, but without CT evidence of disease, should not dictate surgical violation of the ostiomeatal unit.

Frontal Sinus

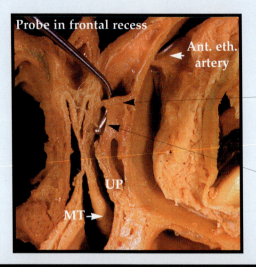

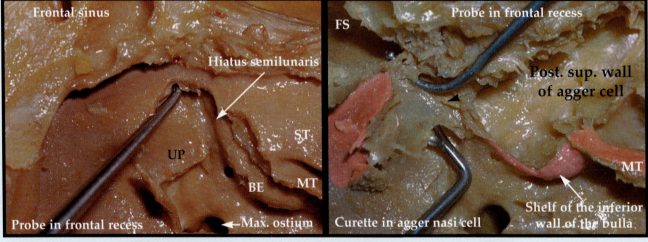

The upper third of the uncinate process merges laterally over the lateral nasal wall, covering the agger nasi cells. Identification of this part is crucial. The space between the uncinate process and the middle turbinate leads the surgeon to the frontal recess in the majority of cases.

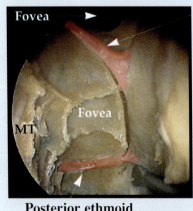

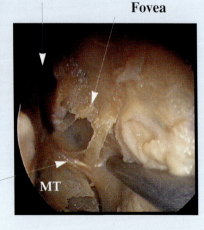

The anterior ethmoid artery enters the nasal cavity at the junction of the fovea and the lamina papyracea. It traverses anteromedially toward the cribriform plate and divides the anterior ethmoid fovea into a smaller anterior and a larger posterior segment. Although the artery is a good landmark in endonasal frontal sinus surgery, contrary to common belief, staying immediately anterior to the artery will lead to the fovea, resulting in disaster. It is therefore important to identify the lacrimal sac and stay along the ascending process of the maxilla and use the course of the artery as a reference point.

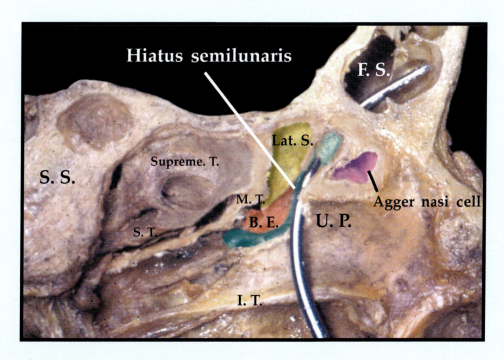

CHARACTERISTICS OF THE FRONTAL SINUS

Development: Develops from pneumatic extension of the anterior ethmoid cells into the frontal bone.
Development begins late in intrauterine life or may start after the birth.

Agenesis: Bilateral—5% (varies from 2% to 35%).
Unilateral—4% (varies from 2.5% to 20%).

Pneumatization & Growth: Occurs from one to twenty years. Pneumatization starts in the vertical segment.

Chambers: Usually two, one on each side.
Three or more chambers in 1.5% to 21% of persons.
Almost always asymmetrical.
Divided by thin bony intrasinus septa, usually off the midline and rarely dehiscent.

Adult Size (Averages):

	Van Alyea	Ritter	Lang
Height (mm)	28	28	24.3 (5-66)
Width (mm)	24	27	29.0 (17-49)
Depth (mm) (Anteroposterior)	20	17	20.5 (10-46.5)

Surgical significance: As is evident, the size varies considerably. The depth is the most important dimension. This should be studied individually on the CT scan. That is the space available for a safe entry into the frontal sinus floor.

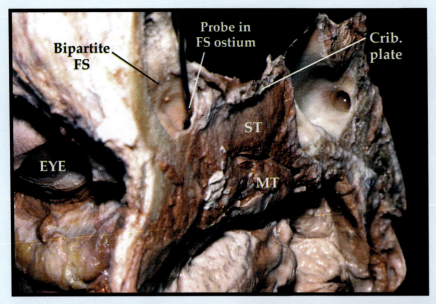

Generally, the frontal sinus has one cavity on each side. Here there are two cavities on the right side. Each cavity has a separate drainage facility. The ostium of the frontal sinus is always situated in the most dependent area of the sinus floor, as seen here. Due to this anatomical fact, frontal sinus infections are less common than infections of other paranasal sinuses.

The light pipe is inserted into the nasal cavity through the frontal sinus opening. Observe the location of the glow of the light, which appears to be in the anteroinferior area of the ethmoid bulla.

The agger nasi cell is the most common and constant cell of the anterior ethmoid. It arises from the lacrimal bone. The number varies from 1 to 3. It drains into the hiatus semilunaris. It is located immediately anterior to the attachment of the middle turbinate.

To reach the frontal sinus endonasally, the surgeon must first resect the agger nasi cell accurately and effectively.

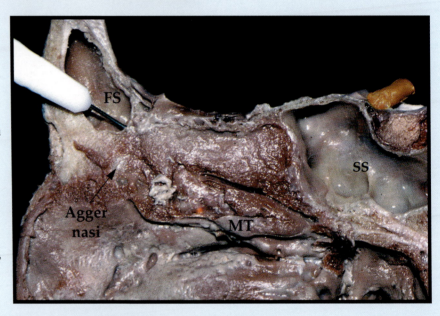

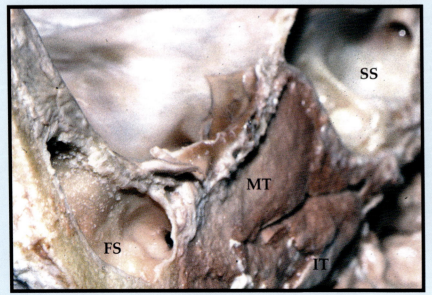

The frontal sinus is pyramidal or funnel shaped, with the apex projected upward.

Surgical significance:
The most common site of injury during the endonasal frontal sinus approach is the junction of the posterior wall of the frontal sinus and the ethmoid fovea posterolaterally and the cribriform plate posteromedially. To avoid this complication, remember to stay anterior and lateral to the attachment of the middle turbinate.

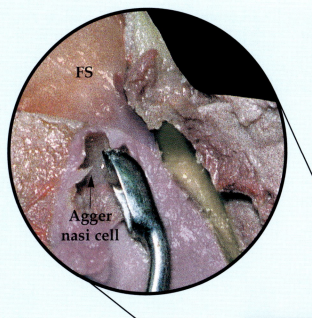

Frontal Recess

The frontal recess is the space where the frontal sinus opens. There are three parts which we should study: the frontal sinus, the ostium and the frontal recess. The first part is the widest; the second part, the nasofrontal isthmus, is the narrowest (the waist); and the third, bottom part, the frontal recess, is somewhat wider. The size and shape of the recess depend on the pneumatization of the agger cells.

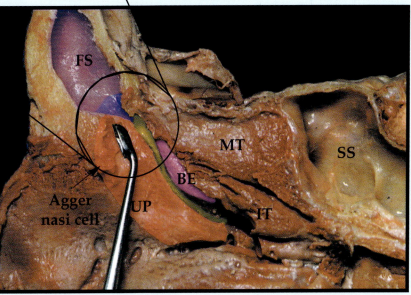

The frontal sinus drains into the frontal recess by a channel. This channel can be very short or it can be long. Lang calls a channel longer than 3 mm a duct, and a shorter channel an ostium.

The size and length of the duct depend on the size, shape and number of pneumatized agger nasi cells. The posterosuperior wall of the agger cell forms the anteroinferior wall of the frontonasal duct and the frontal recess, as seen here.

Surgical significance: We have to study the CT scan to identify the agger nasi cells and their extent. These cells have to be resected in order to reach the area where the frontal sinus drains.

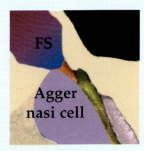

The frontal sinus drains into the hiatus semilunaris. Most commonly the channel enters the hiatus semilunaris in its anterosuperior part, as shown here. However, it can open into the hiatus semilunaris in its posterior part, medially, or occasionally into its lateral segment. Its incidence is 15% (Van Alyea).

Surgical significance: Whenever there is a well-formed hiatus semilunaris, following it superiorly will invariably lead to the frontal sinus opening.

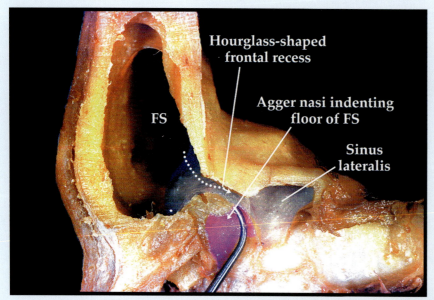

FRONTAL CELLS (FRONTAL BULLA)

The name is given to the ethmoid cells which project into the frontal cavity. Zuckerkandl in 1883 named it "frontal bullae." The reported incidence varies from 8% to 20%.

Here the frontal sinus drains into the lateral sinus. Generally in such cases, the bulla is poorly developed. By following the agger nasi cells methodically, the surgeon can reach the frontal sinus. This kind of drainage system is seen in 1% of cases (Van Alyea).

In the image to the right, the anterior ethmoid cell created a bulge in the floor of the frontal sinus, narrowing the frontal drainage channel.

Surgical significance:
Endonasally it gives the false impression that one has reached the frontal sinus. In reality the surgeon may be in the frontal cell. To reach the frontal sinus and to establish an adequate drainage, the surgeon must resect the superior wall of the frontal cell.

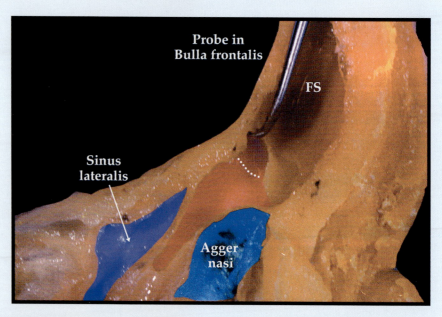

ORBITAL RECESS COURSE

The frontonasal duct opens superiorly, laterally and posteriorly into the lateral sinus. The lateral wall of the frontal recess is bounded by the lamina papyracea. Here also the bullar cell is poorly developed and the hiatus semilunaris ends abruptly in its anterosuperior course (recessus terminalis).

Surgical significance:
Though finding the natural ostium of the frontal sinus is quite difficult, the sinus can be entered endonasally, as described later in the technique.

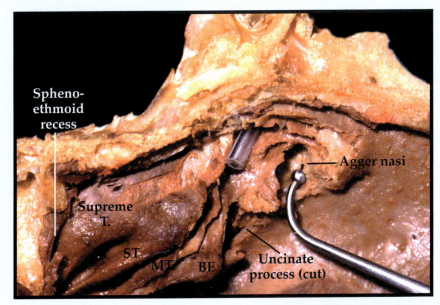

DIRECT MIDDLE MEATUS COURSE

Here, the frontal sinus drains directly into the middle meatus. The bullar cell is small and the hiatus semilunaris is short. It ends anterosuperiorly in a horizontal bony bar. This condition is known as recessus terminalis. The frontal recess is bounded:
- Medially by the lamina of the middle turbinate.
- Laterally by the agger and anterior ethmoid cells.
- Anteriorly by the agger nasi cell.
- Posteriorly by the anterosuperior bullar cells.

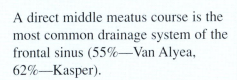

A direct middle meatus course is the most common drainage system of the frontal sinus (55%—Van Alyea, 62%—Kasper).

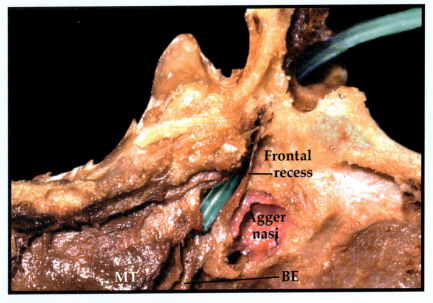

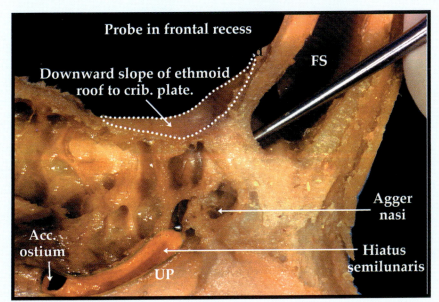

SUPERIOR-LATERAL ENTRANCE INTO THE HIATUS SEMILUNARIS

Here, the frontal sinus drains into the hiatus semilunaris in its superior lateral segment.

Again, observe the agger nasi cells, which are located at the attachment of the middle turbinate and medial to the frontal recess.

SPHENOID SINUS

The sphenoid sinus is a bilateral pneumatization of the sphenoid bone. Symmetry in the two sinuses is unusual. Variations in size, shape, pneumatization, and the number of septa are so common that Van Alyea has regarded variability as "typical of the anatomy of the sphenoid sinus." Congdon describes the sphenoid sinus as "the most variable in form of any bilateral cavity or organ in the human body."

The walls of the sphenoid sinus vary in thickness, depending on its pneumatization. Generally the anterosuperior wall and the roof are the thinnest (0.1 mm to 1.5 mm) and may even show some dehiscence. The anteroinferior wall and the floor are thickest. Intrasphenoidal neural and vascular projections of vital neighboring structures and ridges and recesses in the walls and the floor are characteristics of this sinus.

The sphenoid sinus exhibits wide variation in degree of pneumatization. Pneumatization may extend as far as the clivus, the lesser wing, the anterior clinoid process, the foramen magnum, the foramen lacerum and the occipital bone. Agenesis of the sinus occurs in about 1% of cases.

Types of pneumatization

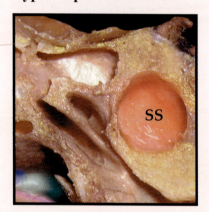

Conchal
0%—Lang
5%—Congdon

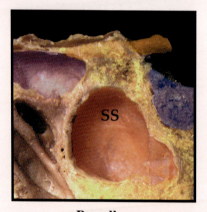

Presellar
23.8%—Lang
28.0%—Congdon

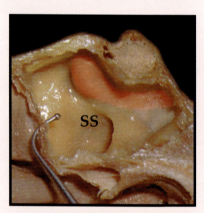

Sellar (including "postsellar")
76.2%—Lang
67.0%—Congdon

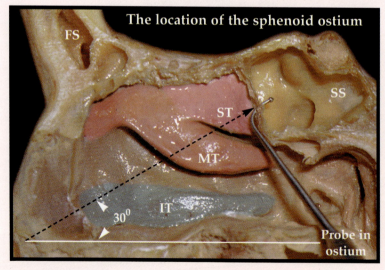

The sphenoid ostium is on a line that makes a 30-degree angle to the floor of the nose at an average distance of 6.5 cm from the nasal spine. However, I have found in cadaveric dissections and surgery that the angle can vary from 30 to 40 degrees. The distance varies in different races. It is largest in African Americans and smallest in Asians. These facts can serve as a guideline in identifying the sphenoid ostium.

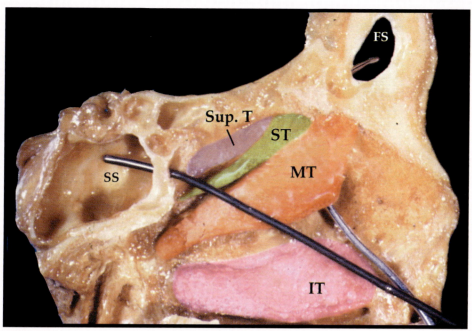

CHARACTERISTICS OF THE SPHENOID SINUS

Development: Develops from a mucosal invagination into the sphenoid bone from the posterosuperior recess of the nasopharynx. Development begins in the third fetal month.

Agenesis: Rare. Rudimentary sinus or conchal pneumatization is seen in approximately 1% of cases.

Pneumatization & Growth: Starts in the third or fourth year and generally ends in the fourteenth year.

Chambers: Usually two, one on each side.
Almost always asymmetrical.
Divided by thin bony intrasinus septa, usually off the midline and occasionally dehiscent or absent. The septa can terminate on the carotid or the optic canal.

Adult Size (Average):

	Van Alyea	Dixon	Lang (center part)
Height (mm)	19.5 (5-33)	18-20	24.3 (5-66)
Width (mm)	17.4 (2.5-34)	15-17	29.0 (17-49)
Depth (mm) (Anteroposterior)	23.2 (4-44)	19-22	20.5 (10-46.5)

Surgical significance:
1. The sphenoid sinus should be entered approximately 1 cm below the fovea as this is the thinnest bony part.
2. Extreme care should be taken to avoid injury to the lateral, posterior and superior walls of the sinus as very important structures lie here (i.e., the cavernous sinus with its contents, internal carotid artery, the pituitary fossa and the brain).
3. Care should be taken while removing the septa of the sphenoid as these may be attached to the carotid or optic canal and injury here may result in death and blindness, respectively.

Intrasphenoid Projections

INTERNAL CAROTID ARTERY

    65%—Van Alyea
    85.7%—Lang

OPTIC NERVE

    40%—Van Alyea
    19%—Lang

MAXILLARY NERVE (V_2)

    40%—Van Alyea
    28.6%—Lang

VIDIAN NERVE

    36%—Van Alyea
    14.3%—Lang

ABDUCENT NERVE

    34%—Van Alyea
    4.8%—Lang

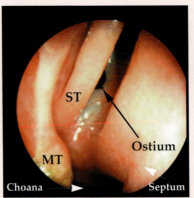

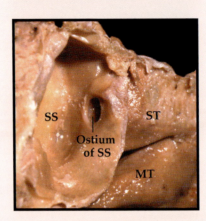

Sphenoid Ostium

Generally:
- Located high in the sphenoethmoid recess.
- Close to the midline in the anterior sphenoid wall at the junction of the upper one-third and lower two-thirds of it (0.6-0.9 mm from the midline, according to Lang).
- A few millimeters from the cribriform plate (Peele).
- Medial to supreme or superior turbinate.
- Round, oval or a vertical cleft.
- 1.0 mm to 5.0 mm in size.

But:
- It can be located anywhere in the anterior wall, from the midpoint to close to the floor. The distance from the floor of the sphenoid sinus to the ostium may vary from 4 to 20 mm.

Supraoptic and Infraoptic Recesses

These recesses are prominent when pneumatization extends into the lesser sphenoid wing.

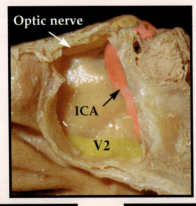
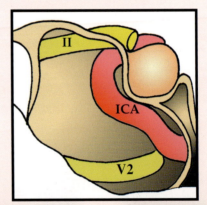
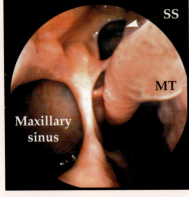
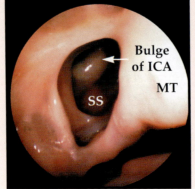
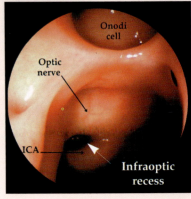

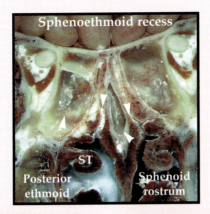

Sphenoid Rostrum

The midline projection of the anterior sphenoid wall. It articulates with the perpendicular plate of the ethmoid and the vomer.

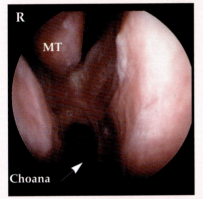
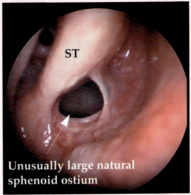

Sphenoethmoid Recess

A space behind and above the most superior turbinate.
It is well formed in over 50% of cases. This space is bounded:
- Posteriorly by the anterior wall of the sphenoid.
- Anterolaterally by the uppermost concha (superior or supreme).
- Medially by the nasal septum.
- Superiorly by the cribriform plate.
- Inferiorly it opens into the nasopharynx.
- Depth varies according to the configuration of the uppermost concha.
- Sphenoid ostium and posterior ethmoid cells.

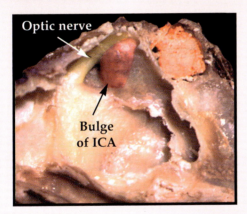

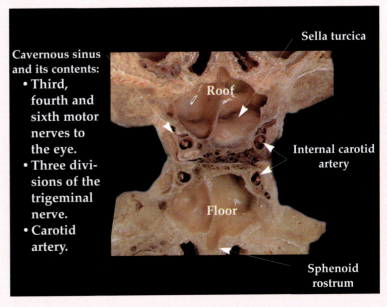

Cavernous sinus and its contents:
- Third, fourth and sixth motor nerves to the eye.
- Three divisions of the trigeminal nerve.
- Carotid artery.

51

4
MINIMALLY INVASIVE TECHNIQUES IN ENDOSCOPIC SINUS SURGERY

"The rhinologist must direct his attention toward the restoration and maintenance of adequate drainage channels, this to be done with the least possible damage to functioning nasal and sinus structure."—Van Alyea.

This principle is as true today as it was in 1945. Have we followed it in the last several years? The number of endoscopic sinus surgical procedures performed in the United States increases every year. Usually these procedures are standard techniques, such as anterior or posterior approach ethmoidectomies performed for minimal or extensive disease. Although endoscopic sinus surgery is in itself a minimally invasive technique, this is so in comparison with the older techniques, e.g., external ethmoidectomy, the Caldwell-Luc procedure, etc. However, even in endoscopic surgery often less is required than is usually done. For instance, removal of the entire uncinate process and anterior ethmoid is too aggressive a procedure for treating limited disease in the ostiomeatal unit. It can result in loss of normal mucosa, excessive scarring and iatrogenic frontal recess obstruction. Scarring due to loss of ciliary lining increases the risk of recurrent infections. Postoperatively, symptoms persist and in some cases even increase. CT shows worsening sinus disease. These patients, who preoperatively had minimal ostiomeatal disease, now become "sinus cripples." Following are a few examples of the damage that can result from over aggressive surgery.

The patient whose scans are shown below underwent functional endoscopic sinus surgery by an expert endoscopic sinus surgeon for "recurrent sinusitis" based on medical history alone, even though the CT scan was essentially unremarkable. Postoperatively symptoms persisted. The one-year postoperative CT scan revealed bilateral chronic maxillary sinusitis that had not been present before. Maxillary endoscopy with dye study revealed a large patent reconstructed middle meatus ostium, markedly thickened mucoperiosteum of the maxillary sinus with poor mucociliary flow and no evidence of accessory ostia. I recommended a nasoantral window and/or a Caldwell-Luc operation, which the patient refused.

Preoperative CT scan

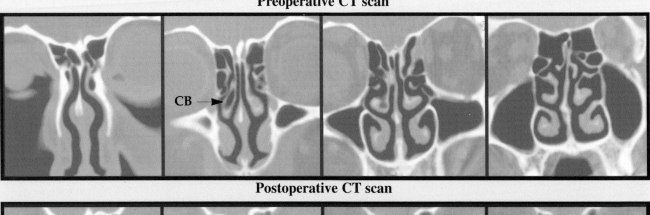

Postoperative CT scan

The young woman whose scans are shown below had inhalant allergies and mild bronchial asthma. Her symptoms included nasal congestion, facial pressure and headache, partially relieved by antibiotic courses. She underwent functional endoscopic sinus surgery with bilateral ethmoidectomy, bilateral maxillary ostium reconstruction, septum reconstruction and turbinate resection. Her postoperative course was a long saga of misery. Her previous symptoms persisted and intensified and new symptoms developed. She complained of left frontal headaches, purulent rhinorrhea, nasal congestion and maxillary pain bilaterally. In my opinion, the surgical procedures performed were overly aggressive in all aspects. Injury to the natural ostium resulted in bilateral maxillary sinusitis. Upper anterior ethmoid cell injury and scarring resulted in frontal sinusitis. The subtotal turbinate resection was excessive. The patient has become a "sinus cripple." Temporary relief is provided by culture-driven prolonged antibiotic courses.

Preoperative CT scan 1993

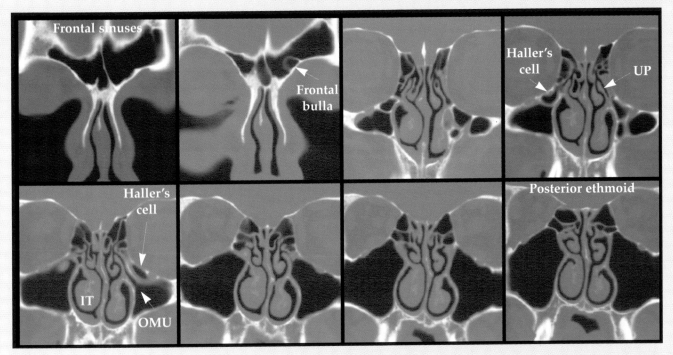

Postoperative CT scan 1994

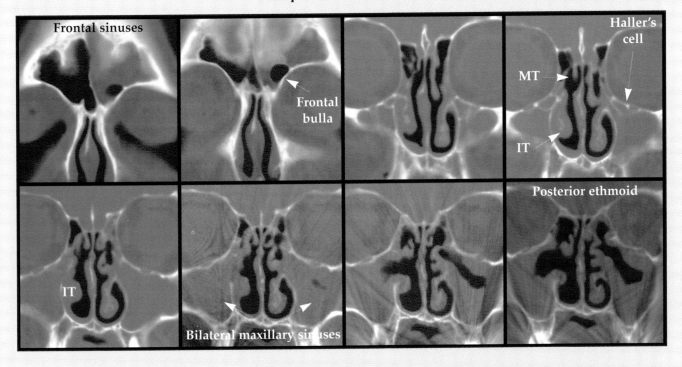

The following patient underwent a bilateral subtotal inferior turbinectomy for chronic nasal congestion. Postoperatively, his symptoms increased, and he had additional complaints of a constant need to clear his nasopharynx, postnasal drip and dryness of the throat. Endoscopic evaluation showed the absence of almost the entire inferior turbinate on both sides and a roomy nose with chronic nasopharyngitis. I could not offer much to this patient.

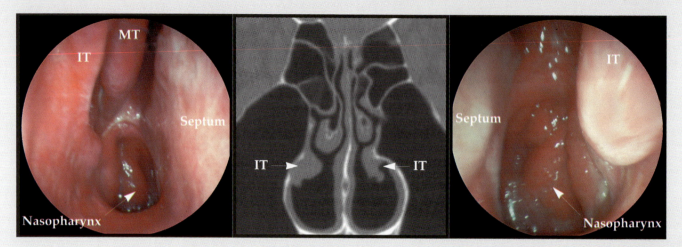

Conclusion

1. Minimal mucosal changes on CT scan do not justify an aggressive approach.

2. Avoid operating on patients based on history alone. The CT scan should show definite abnormality.

3. Avoid manipulating and interfering with the ostiomeatal unit if disease is not evident on CT scan. If obstruction of the ostium is still suspected, perform transcanine maxillary endoscopy and evaluation with dye study before violating a natural ostium.

4. Avoid total or subtotal resection of the turbinates. Reduction turbinoplasty or minimal turbinate surgery is preferable.

Principles of Minimally Invasive Surgery

1. Minimize surgical trauma.
2. Maximize preservation of natural anatomy.
3. Preserve maximum mucosa.
4. Reestablish ventilation.
5. CT scan is the foundation on which surgery should be based. Endoscopic evaluation, though informative, should not be the guiding principle. Surgical steps should be preplanned in relation to the CT scan done during the least symptomatic period.
6. If the disease encountered at surgery is more extensive than anticipated, do not allow it to alter your preplanned surgical decision.
7. Following surgery, enough time should be allowed for normalization of the physiological processes, before considering any further surgery. If the patient is operated on while symptomatic, the disease will seem more virulent than the findings on the CT scan indicate. Ideally, surgery should be deferrred until the patient is relatively symptom free.

All of these goals are attainable only with the advanced techniques and newer instruments that are now available. They also require a thorough knowledge of the anatomy and integration with the CT scan findings.

Our aim is to introduce a new concept of minimally invasive techniques (MIT) for use in endoscopic sinus surgery. Patients with suspected sinus disease are divided into three groups, as shown below. Each group is managed differently. The surgical techniques differ for each group. In our experience, minimally invasive surgical techniques are most beneficial in Groups I and II. In Group III, we apply this concept to avoid complications and reduce recurrence. We have performed these procedures over the past seven years and have refined our techniques with available state-of-the-art technology. This has improved our surgical outcome. Our mission is to carry this message to our colleagues.

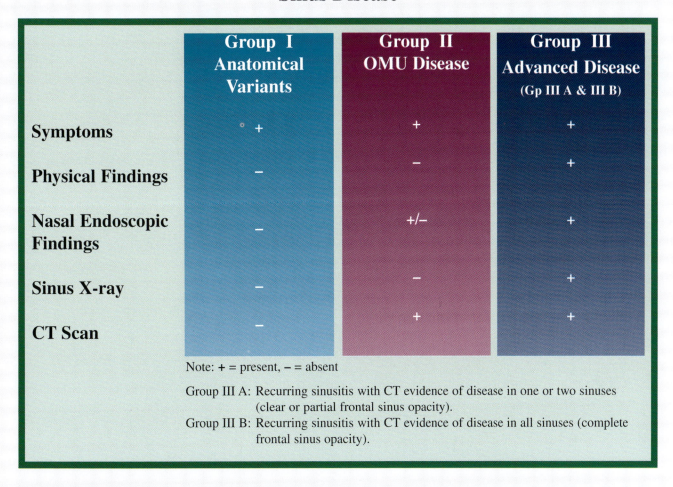

Sinus Disease

	Group I Anatomical Variants	Group II OMU Disease	Group III Advanced Disease (Gp III A & III B)
Symptoms	+	+	+
Physical Findings	−	−	+
Nasal Endoscopic Findings	−	+/−	+
Sinus X-ray	−	−	+
CT Scan	−	+	+

Note: + = present, − = absent

Group III A: Recurring sinusitis with CT evidence of disease in one or two sinuses (clear or partial frontal sinus opacity).

Group III B: Recurring sinusitis with CT evidence of disease in all sinuses (complete frontal sinus opacity).

This book illustrates live surgical procedures in step-by-step continuity. We have used computer-enhanced technology to stress the salient anatomical and surgical features. We hope that this will contribute to improved patient care.

In my eleven years of experience as an endoscopic surgeon, though I cannot claim to have cured 100% of patients, I have not had a single orbital or cranial complication, nor have I had to give a single blood transfusion. I attribute this to four facts: (1) A thorough and precise knowledge of surgical anatomy learned through several cadaveric dissections and teaching courses. (2) Performing minimally invasive surgery, where less is always better than more. (3) Use of the KTP/532 laser. The fineness of its tip (0.6 mm) allows me to make an incision as small as 1 mm. The relatively bloodless field allows good visualization. (4) Use of the microdebrider allows for a good mucosa-sparing technique.

The KTP laser and microdebrider are not available everywhere. Not all surgeons may be comfortable with these instruments. The key point is to make yourself fully aware of all anatomical configurations and use whichever instrument is available or whichever you are comfortable with, carefully and with precision.

INSTRUMENTS

The following instruments are indispensable for the performance of minimally invasive techniques.

All large standard biters should be discarded from the tray and one should invest in small-jaw pediatric forceps, Thru-Cut and Sure-Cut small-jaw forceps.

These instruments are superior to the standard ones. Under normal circumstances more than 50% of cases have a considerable amount of oozing. Use of the standard instruments results in mucosal tearing, increased oozing, obscuring of the surgical field and inadvertent cellular damage. The Thru-Cut forceps, the microdebrider and the KTP/532 laser prevent these events, resulting in a true minimal invasion of tissue.

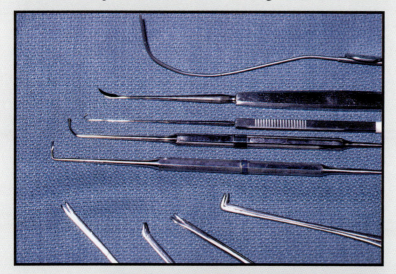

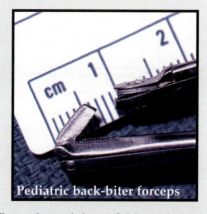

Pediatric back-biter forceps

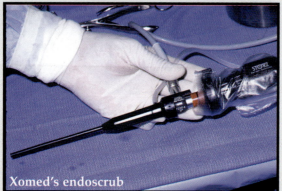

Xomed's endoscrub

The endoscrub is useful in maintaining a clean field, reducing tissue scatter and cooling the surgical area during laser surgery with Ho:YAG or Nd:YAG. However, it has a limitation: it is operated with a foot control. It is not advisable to operate two foot controls at the same time.

I prefer to prepare my own nasal splints using a folded piece of Telfa with a No.18 gauge suction cannula inserted in the fold, to allow ventilation—as shown below.

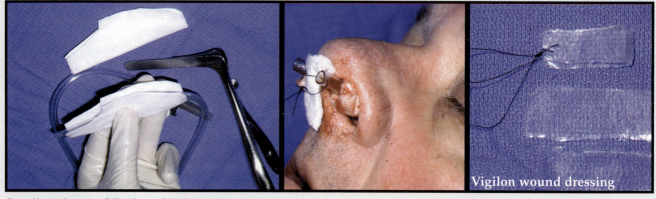

Vigilon wound dressing

Smaller pieces of Telfa or Vigilon can also be used as middle meatal splints. These are economical and well-tolerated by patients.

For adequate exposure of the agger nasi and the frontal recess, the only instrument that works effectively is the power drill. The Fisch power drill, which was introduced to me by Dr. Draf, has a long shaft and a long diamond bur. The positioning of the drill system along the endoscope is very important. Misplacement can damage the endoscope. The diamond bur provides stability and hemostasis and prevents excessive resection.

The recently introduced Xomed's XPS Straightshot Micro Resector System and Linvatec's Apex Shaver System offer the advantage of a dual function. It can be used as a microdebrider and a power drill. A protective sleeve with the 3.5-mm spherical bur makes it especially useful for intranasal dacryocystorhinostomy and frontal sinus surgery.

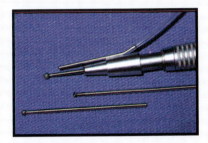
Fisch power drill

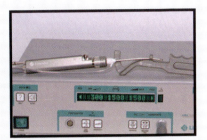
Linvatec Apex Shaver System

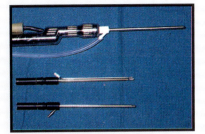
Xomed's XPS Straightshot Micro Resector System

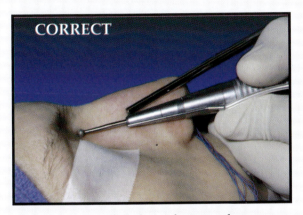
Correct way to align the endoscope along the drill—intranasally.

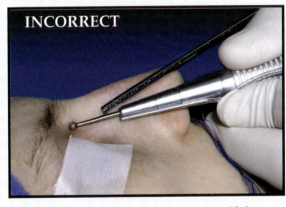
Incorrect way to align the endoscope. If the rotating part of the drill touches the scope, the scope will be damaged.

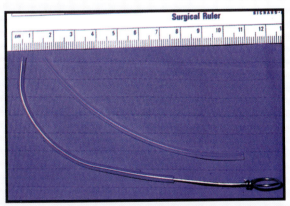

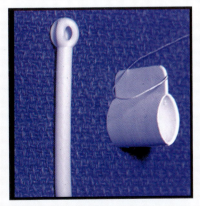

A 10 fr. (1/8") silicone round drain tubing with a stylet inserter can be used to stent the frontal sinus ostium. The tube should be sutured to the nasal septum. On the right are shown commercially available stents for the frontal sinus and the middle meatus.

MICRODEBRIDER

Since the advent of endoscopic sinus surgery in the U.S.A. in 1985, it has become widely recognized that overaggressive surgery results in a less than ideal outcome. The aim has therefore been mucosal sparing and the least possible amount of trauma to the tissues. The introduction of the microdebrider has brought a new dimension to endoscopic sinus surgery. Persistent efforts by Dr. Setliff and Dr. Parsons have resulted in an instrument with refined edges. It is presently marketed by four companies. We have used products of all these companies on numerous surgical cases and found them to be comparable and of good quality.

The microdebrider is a power rotary instrument that in its original form was a TMJ instrument. It has been modified for sinus use after showing promise in that field. It has the advantages of a small diameter and a rounded tip, which reduces trauma to the mucosa. The tip consists of two parts: an outer protective sheath with a window at the end, and a blade (a rotating shaft) in the window that allows resection on only one side, again reducing trauma. The stem of the microdebrider is hollow, providing for suction. The rotating blade should be used in an oscillating manner rather than in one direction. This reduces the chances of damaging the lamina papyracea. Use of this instrument results in mucosal sparing, less traumatic surgery, clear visualization, reduced operating time and faster healing.

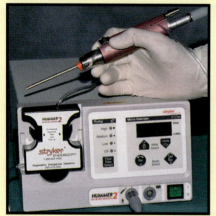

Hummer—ENT Microdebrider 2

A second-generation microdebrider system is offered by Stryker Endoscopy, a Santa Clara, CA, company. Improved suction and irrigation with a disposable irrigation cassette and a speed adjustable to 3000 rpm are its features. The system offers aggressive and jaguar cutters 3.5 mm and 4.0 mm in size.

Linvatec Apex Shaver System

Marketed by Linvatec Corp., a Florida-based company. The key features are:
- Rhinotec blades bendable up to 15 degrees. The bend can be changed many times during the procedure to reach the recesses.
- 3.5-mm and 4.5-mm spherical burs with protective sleeves, at a forward cutting speed of 3000 to 3500 rpm.
- Opening of the cutting window can be rotated 360 degrees in 30-degree increments.
- 3.7-mm and 4.2-mm Cuda and Gator blades.

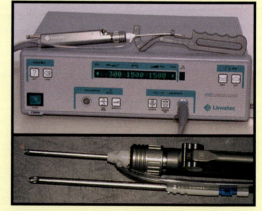

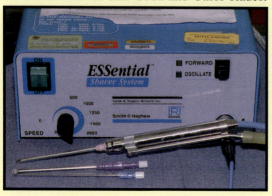

ESSential Sinus Shaver

This microdebrider system is designed and marketed by a Memphis-based company, Smith & Nephew ENT Inc. It has a powerful suction because of an air-tight seal. The handpiece is lightweight and user-friendly. The system provides smooth and serrated blades in 3-mm, 3.5-mm and 4-mm sizes.

Recommended speed for the soft tissue is 1200 rpm and for the ethmoid bone is 2700 rpm.

XPS Straightshot Micro Resector System is a second generation microdebrider by Xomed Surgical Products, Jacksonville, Florida.
- A lightweight (4.7 oz) and powerful handpiece (3000 rpm in oscillation and upto 6000 rpm in rotation).
- Powerful suction with significantly reduced clogging.
- Irrigated blades and burs (2.9-mm to 4.5-mm).
- The multi-function XPS Console allows operation of the Straightshot sinus handpiece, Powerforma high speed mastoid handpiece and Skeeter microdrill.

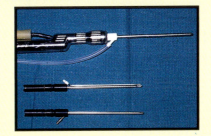

Surgical Technique with the Microdebrider

- Tips: 4.0 mm, 3.5 mm and 2.9 mm are most commonly used.

- Power setting: 1200 rpm to 3000 rpm with oscillating action setting.

Use of the microdebrider is more effective with a clear understanding of the underlying anatomy. It is advisable to gauge the depth of the ethmoid cells before applying the microdebrider. Avoid contact with the bony plates of the lamina papyracea and the skull base and use only oscillating action to prevent any injury. The aim in using the microdebrider is to keep the mucosal lining over the bony plates of vital structures intact and undamaged. This is rather difficult to achieve with the standard instruments.

The following CT sections are at 7.5 mm, 12 mm and 16.5 mm respectively from the nasion.

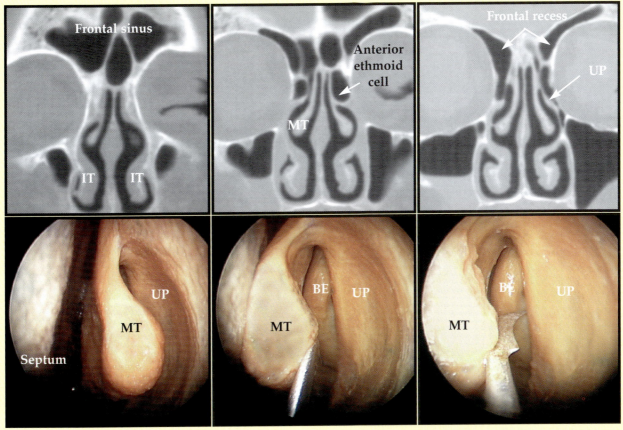

First endoscopic view of the left nasal cavity.

Define the uncinate plate and incise the inferior half of the uncinate process. (Use either a sickle knife or pediatric reverse cutting forceps.)

The following CT sections are at 19.5 mm, 21 mm and 22.5 mm respectively from the nasion.

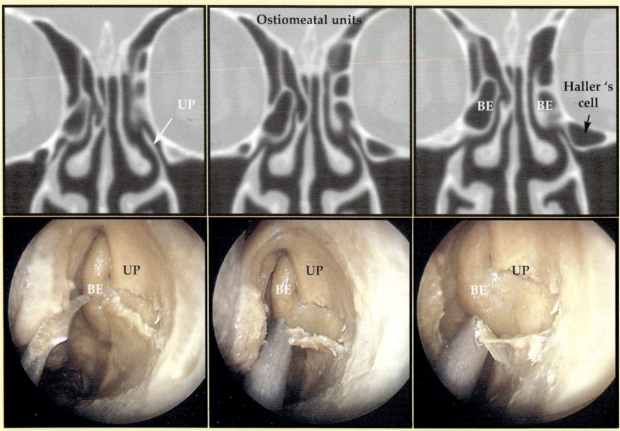

The incised uncinate process provides a good grasping surface for the microdebrider. Avoid injury posterior to the uncinate process.

Use the microdebrider to peel the mucosa off the medial part and the free edge of the uncinate process.

Remove the bony plate of the uncinate process, preserving the inner ostial mucosa.

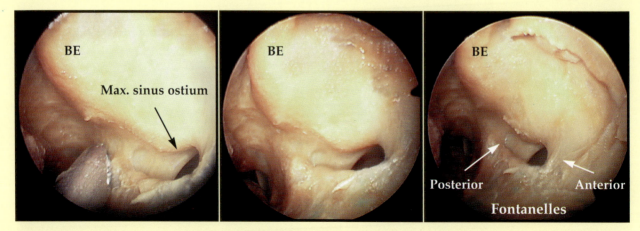

Resect the remaining uncinate process with the microdebrider.

Reconstructed maxillary ostium. If necessary, enlarge the ostium at the expense of the posterior fontanelle, preserving maximal ostial mucosa.

The following CT sections are at 24 mm, 25.5 mm and 27 mm respectively from the nasion.

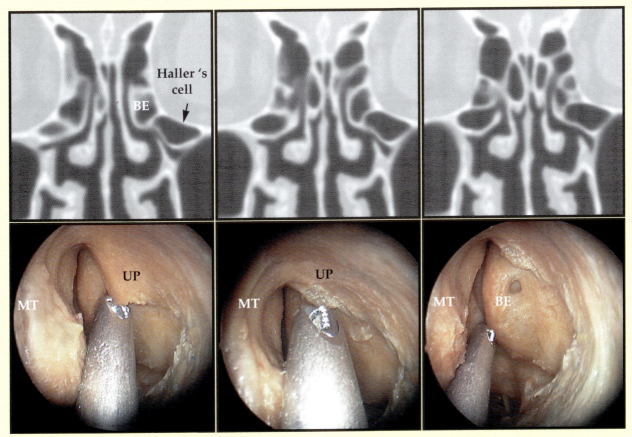

Resect the upper half of the uncinate process without tearing the surrounding mucosa with the microdebrider.

Approach the bulla through the anteroinferior part of its medial wall.

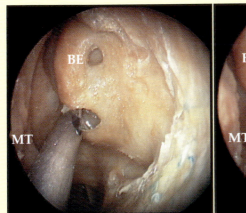

Create a window in the bulla.

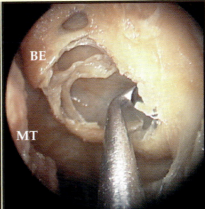

Explore the inner bullar margins with the bent curette.

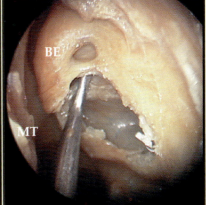

Gauge the overhang of the anterior wall of the bulla by feeling the roof with a blunt probe.

Remove the posterior wall of the bulla.

Observe upper attachment of the bulla to part of the anterior wall.

Remove the anterior wall of the bulla up to its visible superior extent.

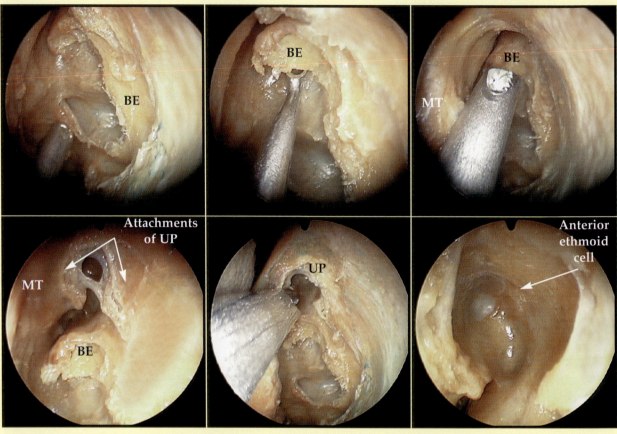

Visualized space is between the upper part of the uncinate process and the anterosuperior bullar wall.

Remove the uncinate process attachments.

Inner view of the anterosuperior ethmoid cell (frontal recess is posterosuperior to this cell).

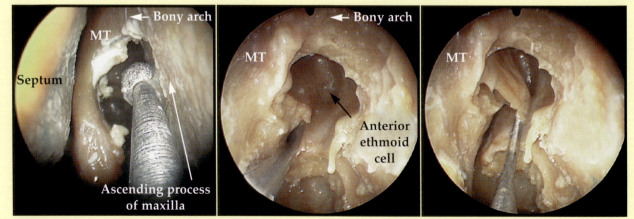

Thin out the ascending process of the maxilla to expose the anterosuperior ethmoid cell. This needs to be done with the power drill. Now the cell is fully exposed.

Separate the medial wall of the cell from the middle turbinate and resect it.

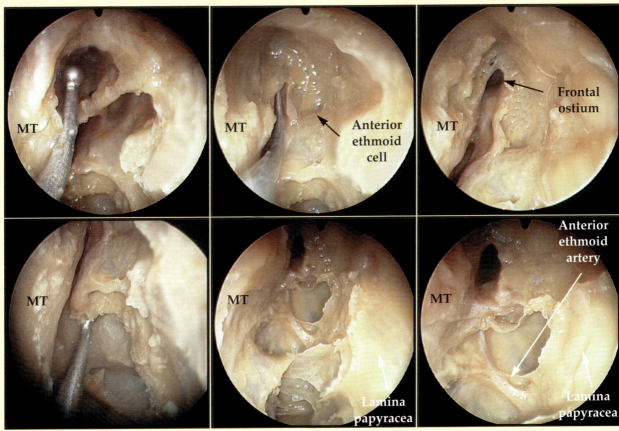

Resect the medial wall of the cell to expose the frontal recess.

Probe in the frontal recess behind the posterosuperior wall.

The frontal sinus ostium.

Remove the suprabullar cells.

Complete the anterior ethmoidectomy and delineate the fovea.

Anterior ethmoid artery in its canal.

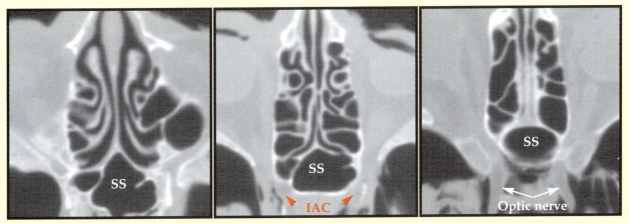

Axial views are indispensable for sphenoid sinus surgery. They should be studied very carefully for the location of the septa and bony dehiscence.

The following CT sections are at 28.5 mm, 31.5 mm and 34.5 mm respectively from the nasion.

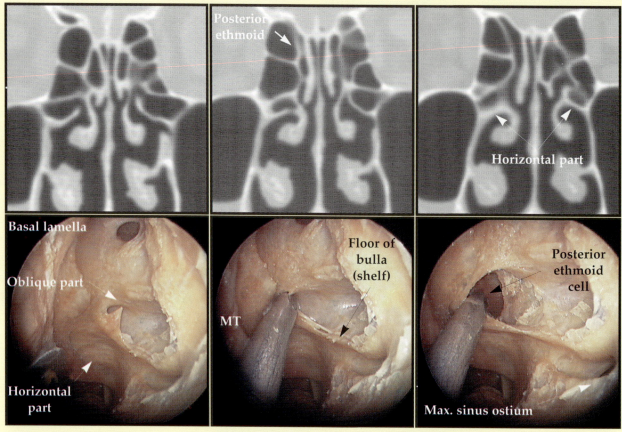

Define the oblique and horizontal parts of the basal lamella.

Approach the posterior ethmoid by perforating the oblique part of the basal lamella just above its junction with the horizontal part.

Continue dissection of the oblique part of the basal lamella using a circumferential hand motion. The microdebrider should always be kept parallel to the inferior border of the middle turbinate and the maxillary ostium.

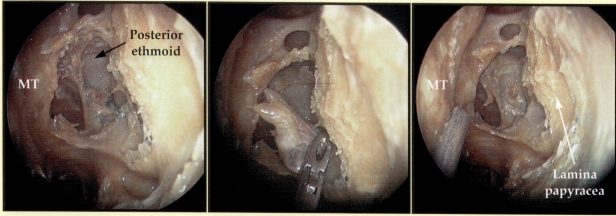

Excise the posterior ethmoid cells.

Remove all visible disease with a cutting forceps or with the microdebrider.

Posterior ethmoid cells.

The following CT sections are at 37.5 mm, 40.5 mm and 43.5 mm respectively from the nasion.

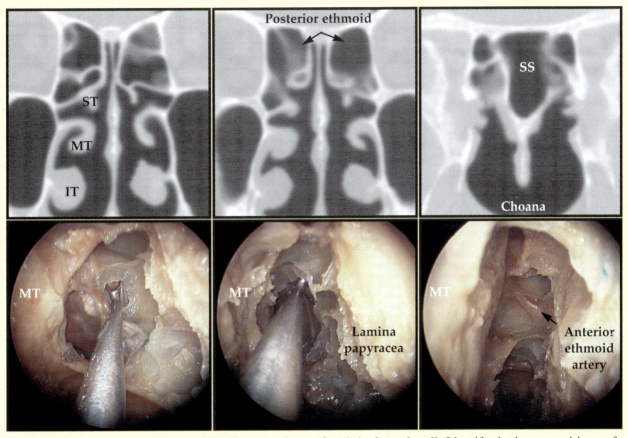

Explore the posteriormost ethmoid cells up to the roof and the lateral wall. Identify the bony partitions of the posterior ethmoidal cells and their overhang and resect them. This step is neccessary to define the skull base. The disease is then resected along the skull base from the posterior to anterior direction.

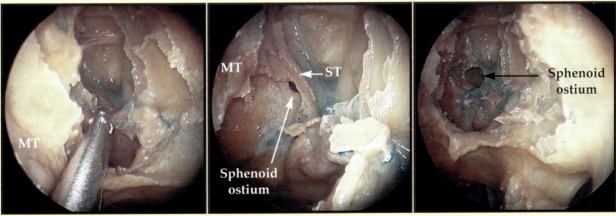

Posteromedial dissection with excision of the superior turbinate to expose the sphenoethmoid recess.

The sphenoethmoid recess exposed, revealing the ostium.

Sphenoid ostium enlarged at the expense of the anterolateral wall.

65

LASERS

There are several lasers on the market. The million-dollar question is, Which is the ideal laser?

Technological developments in lasers and their delivery systems have accelerated in the last decade with renewed interest and enthusiasm. At our institute (Sherman Hospital), we have two CO_2, two KTP/532, one neodymium:YAG, and one holmium:YAG laser, and various other ophthalmological lasers.

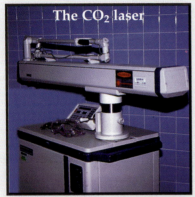

The CO_2 laser

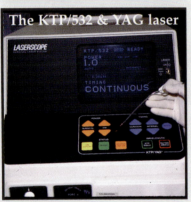

The KTP/532 & YAG laser

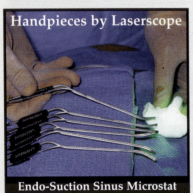

Handpieces by Laserscope

Endo-Suction Sinus Microstat

I was introduced to the world of lasers in 1975 by Dr. Albert Andrews at the Eye and Ear Infirmary, University of Illinois at Chicago. Since then I have tried and tested almost all the lasers that have come on the market. The CO_2 laser is nonflexible (it is semirigid), which makes it less maneuverable and hence limits the structures that are accessible to it in rhinological surgery. Moreover, the CO_2 laser cannot be used in a contact mode and has a poor coagulative effect.

The argon laser does not have a good delivery system nor does it have enough power for rhinological surgery.

The Nd:YAG laser can be used for turbinate and middle meatus reconstruction procedures in a contact technique. However, this laser is quite cumbersome to use either with the sapphire tip or with the bare fiber. It is associated with marked thermal reaction requiring continuous water or warm saline irrigation. This water immersion technique is called "hydrolasing." Its cutting effect is less than optimum, and access to the uncinate plate, maxillary ostium and sphenoethmoid recess is extremely limited.

The holmium laser is a pulsed, high-power laser that causes minimal thermal damage to tissue with almost no charring, provided it is used under water. When not used under a fluid medium, it has an obnoxious effect. The tissue explodes like mini-bombs, spattering the endoscope and making a mess. This obscures the surgical field tremendously and in a split second one can injure tissue that may not have been targeted, or injure the lamina papyracea. The other characteristic of this laser is that it has a pulse action accompanied by a machine gun-like noise, as opposed to a desirable smooth, air brush-like action. In spite of this, one can use the Ho:YAG laser in rhinology with caution. The tissue must be bathed with water while the laser is being applied. The Nd:YAG laser can be used in a similar manner.

I started using the KTP/532 laser in 1987, and found myself becoming partial to it and using it more and more frequently. I now use it exclusively for almost all procedures in rhinology. By keeping the power constant and varying the working distance between the tip and the tissue, the surgeon can achieve coagulation, vaporization and a cutting effect with this laser. The trick is to learn how and where to apply the laser energy. To maintain objectivity and impartiality, I performed comparative studies of the KTP/532 with the other lasers, e.g., Ho:YAG, Nd:YAG, etc. At least 25 cases were performed for each laser studied, where one side was done with the KTP/532 laser and the other with the laser being studied. Hence, my opinions stated throughout this book regarding the various lasers are based on actual use and experience with all of these lasers. Although minimally invasive surgery can also be satisfactorily performed with the newer non-laser instruments that are now available, such as the mucosa-sparing forceps and the microdebrider, optimal finesse is possible only with the KTP laser.

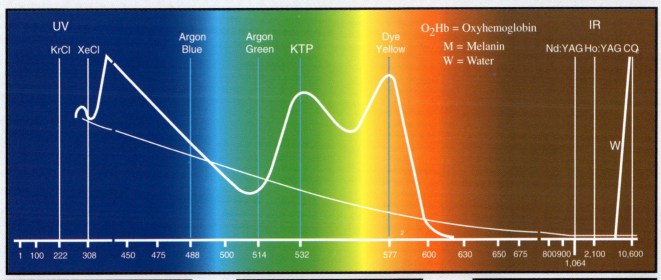

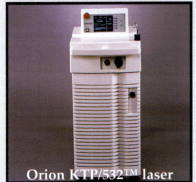
Orion KTP/532™ laser

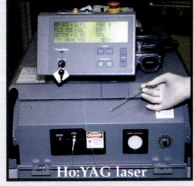
Ho:YAG laser

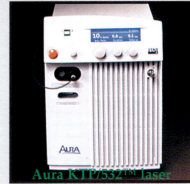
Aura KTP/532™ laser

Surgical Lasers

	KTP/532	Nd:YAG	Ho:YAG	CO$_2$
Wavelength	532	1064	2140	10600
Active Medium	Neodymium in yttrium-aluminum-garnet	Neodymium in yttrium-aluminum-garnet	Holmium in yttrium-aluminum-garnet	CO$_2$, N$_2$, & He gas mixture
Excitation Source	Flash-lamp	Flash-lamp	Flash-lamp	DC discharge or RF discharge
Power Range	< 1 to 40	< 1 to > 100	< 1 to 80	< 1 to > 100
Absorption Length	2 - 3 mm	3 - 4 mm	0.5 mm	0.02 mm
Absorbing Chromophore	Hemoglobin, melanin	Dark-colored tissue	Water	Water

Application of Laser Systems in Endoscopic Sinus Surgery: A Comparative Study

Laser System	Limiting Feature	Adaptive Device	Handpieces	Access (Surg. site)	Hemostasis	Precision
KTP/532	Colored glasses	Safety filter	Excellent	Excellent	Excellent	Excellent
Nd:YAG	Prolonged heat	Hydroscopic	Poor	Fair	Very good	Good
Ho:YAG	Splatter	Endoscrub	Poor	Good	Excellent	Very good
CO$_2$	Articulating arm	Hollow wave guide	Poor	Poor	Poor	Poor

LASER SETUP

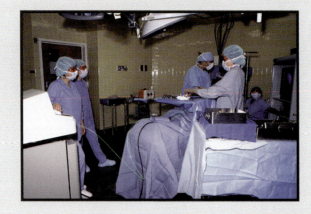

Laser surgery is a team procedure. The team consists of the laser operator, the OR technician, who should have a genuine interest in laser surgery, the circulating nurse and the surgeon. Each contributes equally to a successful outcome. The rule of thumb is that all individuals within eight feet of the laser should wear protective eyeglasses. The laser nurse should be able to adequately visualize the fiber at all times.

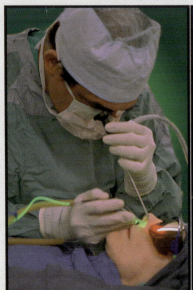

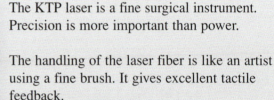

The KTP laser is a fine surgical instrument. Precision is more important than power.

The handling of the laser fiber is like an artist using a fine brush. It gives excellent tactile feedback.

Most of the time, a 0-degree endoscope should be used. It should always be kept parallel to the floor of the nose so that one can visualize the inferior surface of the middle turbinate. The laser delivery device should be kept on the same plane as the endoscope.

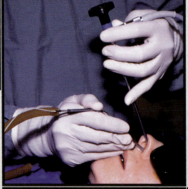

Note hand positions. Holding the scope and the laser delivery device in this manner allows accurate and safe delivery of laser energy.

Careful laser use can avoid potential hazards such as electrical shock, fire, eye injury and skin injury.

During the procedure, it is important to announce "laser standby" and "laser ready."

Eye protection is the number one priority in patient safety, both in local and general anesthesia.

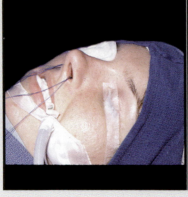
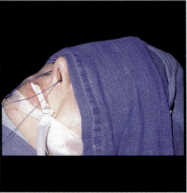

LASER-TISSUE INTERACTIONS

*A Surgical Laser Is an
Instrument That Can Cut, Coagulate and Vaporize*

There are two basic ways to deliver the laser light to tissue: by articulated arms and/or hollow metal tube and by fiberoptic waveguides. The KTP/532 laser is a true fiberoptic laser.

Fiberoptics are flexible and cannot be misaligned. They provide the greatest access to remote tissue sites because of their small size. Light from a fiberoptic diverges as it moves away from the fiber tip. The spot size will increase about 1 mm in diameter for each 4 mm the fiber is moved from the tissue.

Any light that hits tissue will produce a combination of four effects: reflection, absorption, refraction and scatter. The combination of these four effects results in the conversion of light energy into heat energy. Of all these effects, scatter is the most important. The light scatters, or bounces, around the tissue until it is eventually absorbed.

The carbon dioxide and Ho:YAG lasers produce the least scatter, the Nd:YAG the most. The KTP/532 and argon lasers are in between. If there is no scatter, there is no lateral thermal damage and hence no hemostasis. The KTP/532 laser produces a nearly ideal amount of hemostasis for most surgical applications.

When a bare fiberoptic is used in contact it will usually produce a cutting effect. When backed away slightly so that it is in near contact, the effect is mostly vaporization. When moved into a totally noncontact mode, the effect is purely coagulation.

Only the laser foot switch should be kept in the field. All other pedals, including those for the electrocautery and the power drill, should be kept out of the field, so as not to confuse one pedal with the other and cause accidental injury.

When tissue is vaporized, some of the heat that produces the vaporization dissipates into the tissue, producing lateral thermal damage in the form of necrosis and coagulation.

Surgical dosage is described in terms of the amount of laser power delivered, the length of time it is delivered and the size of the exposed area of tissue.

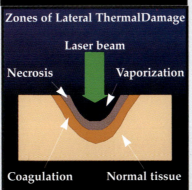

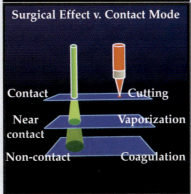

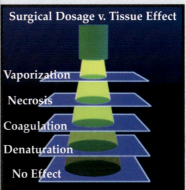

5
SURGICAL TECHNIQUES FOR TURBINATES AND ANATOMICAL VARIANTS (Group I)

Patients in this group pose a challenge. The physical findings are minimal and limited to the turbinates. Endoscopic and CT evaluations are negative for sinus disease, although they may show some anatomical variations. These patients are categorized as having turbinate dysfunction and need to be evaluated further. Most of them should undergo allergy investigation. If positive, as shown in the graphics, treat them, and if they improve, continue with conservative treatment. Those patients who test negative for allergies and those who test positive but do not respond to treatment over a period of six months can be considered for turbinate surgery. They should be endoscopically evaluated in the acute and quiet phases and with and without decongestants before surgery. This makes the selection process more accurate.

Indications for Turbinate Surgery

1. Chronic rhinopathy:
   1. Allergic, cholinergic, reflex.
   2. Chemical, endocrine, synadrenergic, idiopathic.
   3. Mixed.

2. Turbinate disorder leading to ostiomeatal unit obstruction:
   1. Hypertrophic concha.
   2. Concha bullosa.
   3. Paradoxical middle turbinate.
   4. Lateralized middle turbinate.

3. Turbinate surgery to avoid mucosal contact:
   1. Pneumatic large uncinate process.
   2. Pneumatic large bulla ethmoidalis.

4. Turbinate surgery as an adjunct to septal surgery and in patients with narrow noses undergoing aesthetic rhinoplasty.

5. Turbinate surgery as an adjunct to functional endoscopic sinus surgery to help avoid fracture of the middle turbinate and facilitate the approach to the ostiomeatal unit.

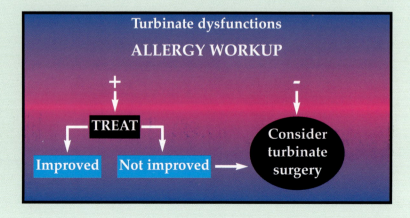

Objective in Turbinate Surgery

Why preserve the turbinates?

"The mucosa has a great ability to regenerate if it is destroyed either by infection, injury, chemicals, or surgery. Regenerated mucosa, however, is less well endowed with cilia and mucous glands and contains scar, which are factors that lessen its resistance to future infections."—Ritter.

The turbinates have a definite physiological function. Care should be taken not to remove them inadvertently. Patients who have undergone resection of a turbinate continue to complain of nasal obstruction, crusting and dryness in the nose. Some also complain of a decreased sense of smell. Turbinate surgery performed with a knife, scissors, freer or cutters invariably results in more resection than planned. It is associated with a higher incidence of intraoperative and postoperative bleeding and synechiae. Nasal packing is required, which increases patient discomfort. The electrocautery is also not suitable for these cases. Following are techniques for inferior and middle turbinate surgery.

Techniques of Inferior Turbinate Surgery

Multiple Island Technique

This is a procedure that I have devised and used for the last 10 years. Three or more vaporization islands are created on the inferior turbinate, depending on the amount of hypertrophy. This is performed with the fiberoptic, flexible KTP/532 laser under direct endoscopic visual control. The size of the islands varies from 1 to 1.5 cm. During resection if the bone is exposed, it should be nibbled off with the Thru-Cut forceps, allowing the soft tissue to overlap the exposed bone. This facilitates healing.

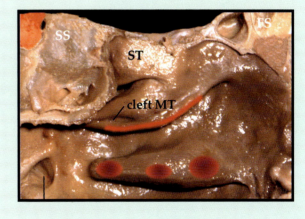

I find the results with this method most consistent and gratifying. This is so because:
(1) There is full visual control of the tissue resection.
(2) The resection is precise and tailored to the amount of turbinate hypertrophy.
(3) The entire turbinate is treated symmetrically, leaving plenty of normal mucosa in between the islands, which results in symmetrical reduction of the inferior turbinate.
(4) The KTP laser provides an almost bloodless field.

The first step after achieving satisfactory anesthesia is to outfracture the inferior turbinate just posterior to the ascending process of the maxilla.

Here, a mulberry-shaped posteroinferior end of the inferior turbinate is vaporized with the KTP/532 laser. Ten watts of laser energy is delivered in a near-contact mode.
As much as one-third of the soft tissue mass can be removed, as seen here.

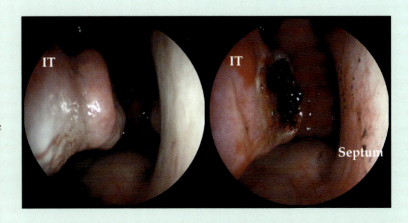

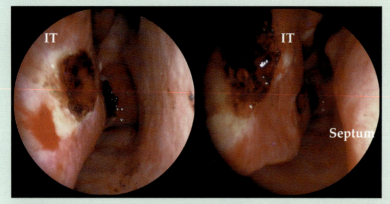

The second island is created in the midportion of the turbinate and the third at the anteroinferior end. This surgery is least traumatic and most precise. One can create more than three islands, depending on the amount of hypertrophy. Plenty of normal tissue should be left in between the islands. This facilitates symmetrical contracture and reduction in the size of the turbinate.

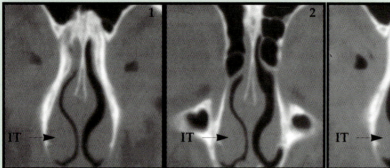
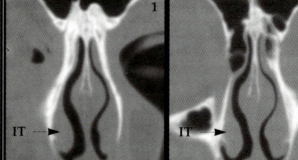

Preoperative CT scan **Postoperative CT scan**

Stripes with Cross-Hatching Technique

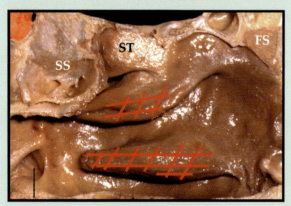

This technique was popularized by Dr. Howard Levine. Two or four stripes are made on the inferior turbinate and if possible on the middle turbinate. These are cross-hatched, as shown here. Care should be taken to leave normal tissue between the crosshatches.

The KTP/532 laser is used at 9 watts of power either in continuous or pulse mode (0.1 sec exposure every 0.1 sec). The near-contact mode is better suited to perform the procedure with excellent hemostasis. Nasal packing is not necessary in the majority of cases.

As you can see here, we are creating stripes across the entire length of the turbinate from the posterior to the anterior end, keeping the laser in an almost contact mode. The depth of the laser burn is approximately 2-3 mm. Generally, two or three stripes are sufficient. Occasionally more may be needed if there is massive hypertrophy. Sufficient normal tissue should be present between the stripes. The stripes are then cross-hatched.

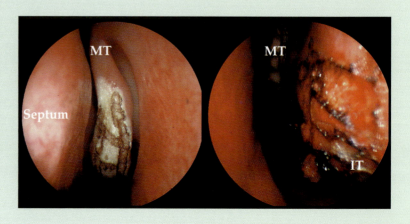

Laser Turbinotomy (Submucous Laser Turbinotomy)

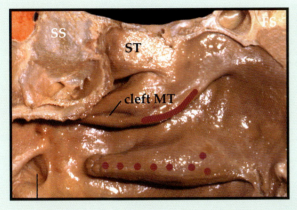

Various techniques have been used to reduce the size of the inferior turbinate. The following technique was devised and is currently used by the author. It requires practice and experience to obtain persistently good results. It is therefore preferable to start with the island technique.

1. After local anesthesia, the inferior turbinate is outfractured.

2. The posterior end of the inferior turbinate is punctured with the KTP/532 laser fiber by firing the laser at 12 watts of power in the pulse mode for 0.1 second every 0.1 second.

3. Laser treatment is given at the periosteal level of the turbinate.

4. The amount of energy needed depends on the bulk of the soft tissue and the underlying bony frame.

5. The tissue reaction should be observed as the laser energy is delivered. The aim is to cause minimal tissue shrinkage during the procedure. This ensures insignificant postoperative crusting.

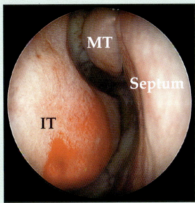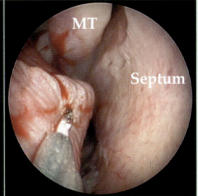

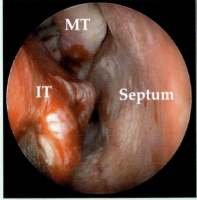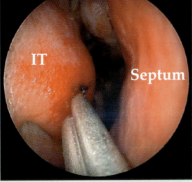

6. At each treatment site, a single entry hole is made on the soft tissue surface of the turbinate. When the bone is reached, a few more holes are made on the turbinate bone with a to-and-fro motion.

7. Depending on the condition and the size of the turbinate, four to eight areas are selected for laser treatment.

Advantages:
- Generally no packing required.
- Minimal bleeding.
- Precise control of tissue depth for laser treatment.
- Maximum preservation of functioning mucosa.
- Less likelihood of adhesion formation.
- Rewarding results.

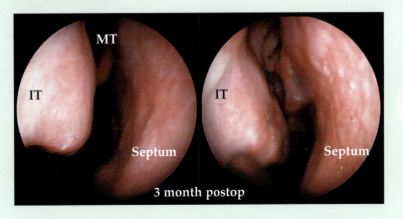

3 month postop

Middle Meatus Obstructive Syndrome (MMOS)

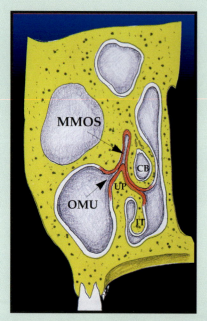

Patients with this disease entity usually present with congestion, facial pressure, nasal obstruction, and postnasal drainage recurring 4 to 10 times per year. Minor head colds and allergic reactions may accompany the above symptoms. They respond well to antibiotics, decongestants and steroid inhalants. CT scans done during symptom-free periods may be normal, may show clouding of the middle meatus and/or may show some anatomical variants such as a large bony concha, concha bullosa, paradoxical middle turbinate, lateralized middle turbinate, large uncinate process or pneumatic large bulla ethmoidalis. This is called middle meatal obstructive syndrome.

Endoscopy, with or without decongestant spray, helps to evaluate the general condition of the turbinates and the middle meatal space. In cases where the turbinates are laterally plastered, the septum is markedly deviated, or the middle turbinate is hypertrophic, evaluation of the ostiomeatal unit is far from satisfactory. In such instances, mucosal edema, contact mucosal polyps, etc., are visualized during the surgical procedure. When the CT scan does not reveal any specific pathology, middle meatus reconstruction and nasal airway reconstruction is planned.

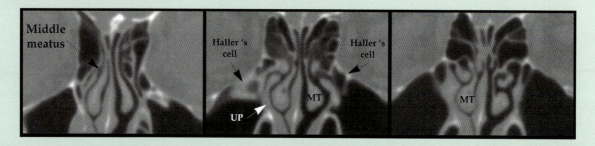

Middle Meatus Reconstruction (MMR)

There are two methods of reconstructing the middle meatus—middle turbinotomy and middle turbinoplasty.

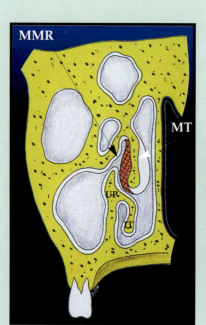

I. Middle Turbinotomy

Precise sculpturing of the middle turbinate with middle meatal reconstruction is an art. The lateral part of the middle turbinate, which faces the lateral wall of the nose, is resected sufficiently to ventilate the middle meatus. This is the easier of the two methods. In the case of concha bullosa, precise excision of the lateral half of the conchal cell is performed. In a hypertrophic turbinate,

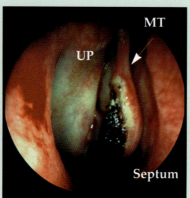

resecting a small segment of the hypertrophic part facing the middle meatus is adequate. Unfortunately, this is difficult to do with the routinely available instruments. Very frequently during the sculpturing, there is injury to the lateral wall, and the middle turbinate ends up being subtotally resected. This excessive resection of the middle turbinate can result in excessive crusting. This can be avoided with the use of the laser, which is more precise in action.

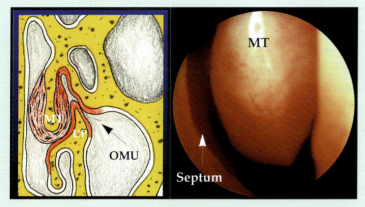

Hypertrophic Concha

This entity presents a special problem. Clinically it may appear to be a case of concha bullosa. However, the CT scan reveals a hypertrophic middle turbinate with crowding of the middle meatus. These cases respond well to middle meatus reconstruction.

A 32-year-old woman presented with recurring left facial pain and headaches. The CT scan revealed a few focal areas of clouding in the ethmoid cells and a hypertrophic turbinate.

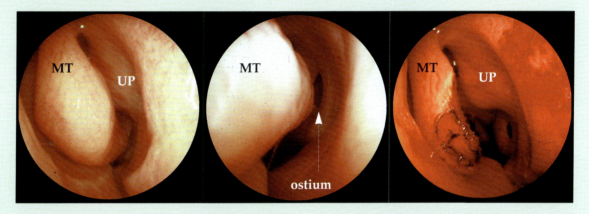

The endoscopic evaluation at surgery revealed crowding of the middle meatus by a protruding, hypertrophic turbinate. This intimate contact of the turbinate with the lateral wall and its protrusion into the accessory ostium were causing the rhinogenic headaches. This was corrected by sculpturing of the middle turbinate, as shown here. The procedure resulted in improved ventilation of the middle meatus, thus alleviating the symptoms. Seven years later, she is still symptom free.

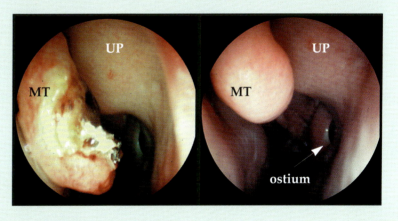

Lateralized Concha

A lateralized middle turbinate that compromises the ostiomeatal unit causes recurring sinusitis. In this case, the right ostiomeatal unit is compromised. A minimal part of the middle turbinate needs to be sculptured, just enough to keep the entire hiatus semilunaris unobstructed. Precise excision with excellent hemostasis is possible with the laser technique. Septum deviation, if present, has to be corrected before the middle turbinate can be sculptured adequately.

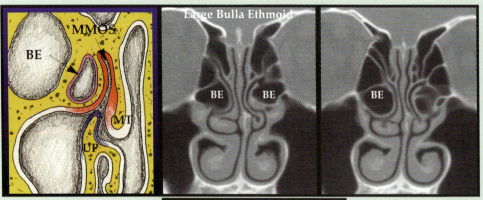

Large Pneumatic Bulla Ethmoidalis

The middle turbinate is sculptured to avoid mucosal contact between the bulla and the lateral surface of the middle turbinate. This technique preserves most of the anterior part of the middle turbinate and ventilates the middle meatus.

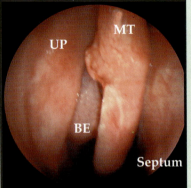

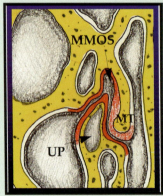
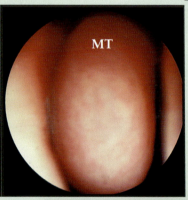

Large Pneumatic Uncinate Process

Here the middle meatus is reconstructed at the expense of the anterolateral segment of the middle turbinate.

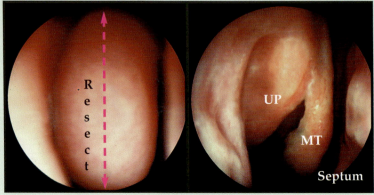

Concha Bullosa

There are two techniques to correct the obstruction created by the concha bullosa: (1) partial conchal resection and (2) conchoplasty.

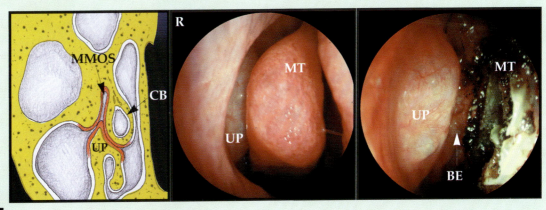

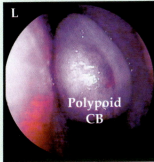

Partial Conchal Resection

The lateral part of the middle turbinate, which faces the ostiomeatal complex, is resected in an adequate amount to reconstruct the middle meatus.

Precise excision of the lateral lamina of the concha bullosa, without fracturing the delicate superior attachment of the middle turbinate, is difficult to accomplish with the standard available instruments, including the Thru-Cut forceps and the microdebrider. With the KTP laser precise excision is possible in almost all cases.

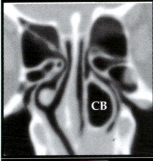

First outline the incision line in a coagulation mode with 9 to 13 watts of power. This also achieves hemostasis. Next, the near-contact mode is used to vaporize the mucosa until the bony lamina is seen and identified. Then, use the laser in the contact mode to cut the thin bony lamella of the concha bullosa. Care should be taken to avoid lateral thermal injury to the mucosa of the medial wall of the concha bullosa, the uncinate process and the bulla ethmoidalis. Gently separate the lateral lamina and remove it. Then evaluate the entire hiatus semilunaris for obstruction. It is of utmost importance not to fracture the superior lamina or superior attachment of the middle turbinate.

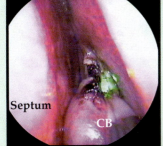

The exposed bone is gently nibbled off and removed. The mucosa is then draped over to cover the exposed bony ridge. Antibiotic ointment is applied over the raw surface.

The second case illustrates step-by-step resection of the lateral lamina of the concha bullosa.

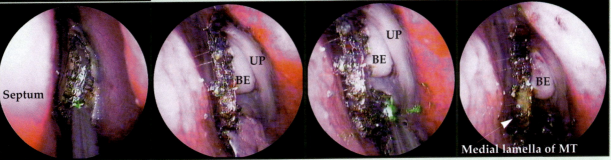

II. Middle Turbinoplasty

After gaining experience in the turbinotomy technique, the surgeon may then advance to the more refined procedures of turbinoplasty and conchoplasty with middle meatus reconstruction. The principle here is maximum mucosal preservation with correction of underlying anatomical defects. An incision is made on the inferior surface of the turbinate mucosa and a subperiosteal flap is created. A part of the turbinate bone is either resected or repositioned, depending on the pathology. The subperiosteal flap is then draped back. This method hastens the healing process, prevents excessive crusting, and improves the physiological functions.

Advantages of middle turbinoplasty
1. Preservation of the anatomical landmark.
2. Preservation of the physiology of mucociliary transport.
3. Avoidance of adhesion and lateralization.
4. Rapid healing.
5. Less crusting and decreased intraoperative and postoperative bleeding.
6. Reduction of crowding and improvement in the ventilation of the middle meatus.

The following is an example of the importance of minimally invasive surgery. A young man complained of recurring nasal congestion, diffuse bilateral facial pressure and a lingering cold. Rhinological examination identified a deviated nasal septum and hypertrophic turbinates. Cultures of the middle meatus were consistently negative. RAST allergy testing was negative. The CT scan below shows a classic case of anterior ethmoid disease. Whenever there is disparity between the symptoms and the CT scan findings, it is wise to take a minimally invasive route. In this case bilateral middle meatus reconstruction, inferior turbinotomy and nasal septum reconstruction were performed. This resulted in complete resolution of the symptoms as well as the CT findings, as is evident in the one-year postoperative CT scan below.

Preoperative CT scan 1995

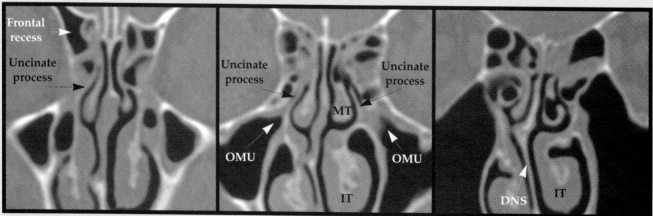

Postoperative CT scan 1996

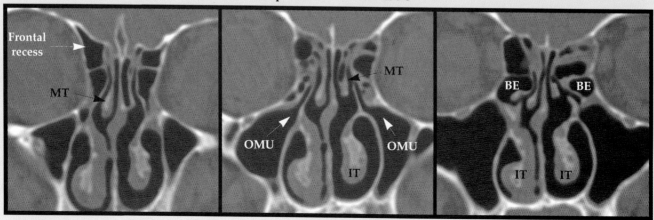

Middle Turbinoplasty

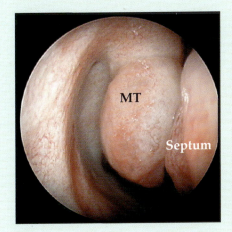

Right paradoxical concha.

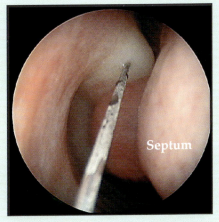

Inject at the junction of the middle turbinate with the lateral wall.

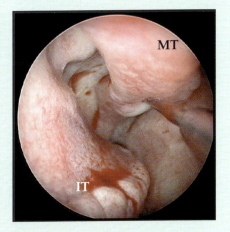

Inject the posterior end of the middle turbinate close to its junction with the lateral wall.

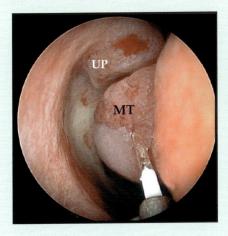

Mucosal incision with use of the KTP laser at 10 to 12 watts of power.

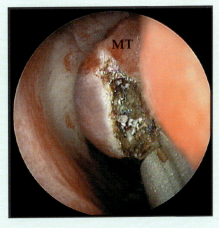

Laser application to the turbinate bone.

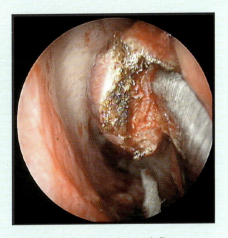

Elevation of subperiosteal flaps.

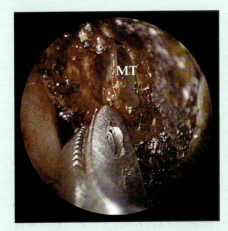

Removal of adequate part of the bone with the Thru-Cut forceps.

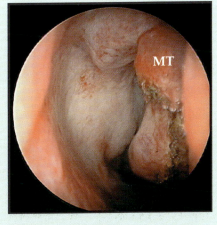

Draping of the subperiosteal flap on the medial bony lamella and evaluation of middle meatus.

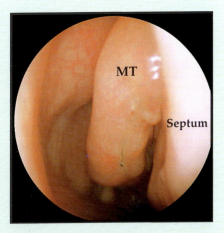

Postoperative view.

Lateralized Concha

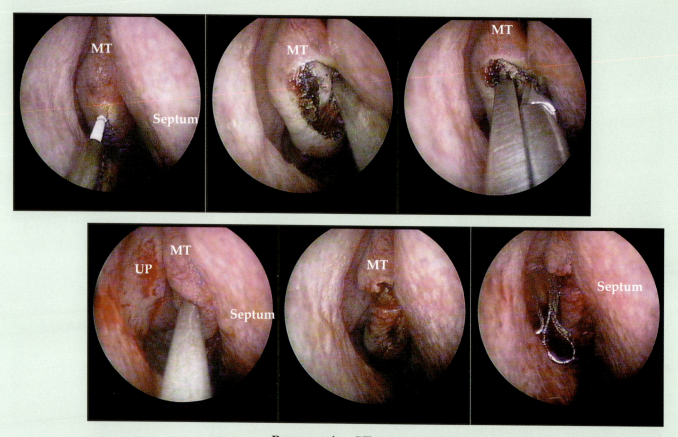

Preoperative CT scan

This patient presented with bilateral middle meatus crowding with lateralized middle concha and bilateral inferior turbinate hypertrophy. Incidental findings included bilateral Haller's cells with a narrow and deep infundibulum. The postoperative CT scan shows improved ventilation of the middle meatus and symmetrical reduction of the inferior turbinates.

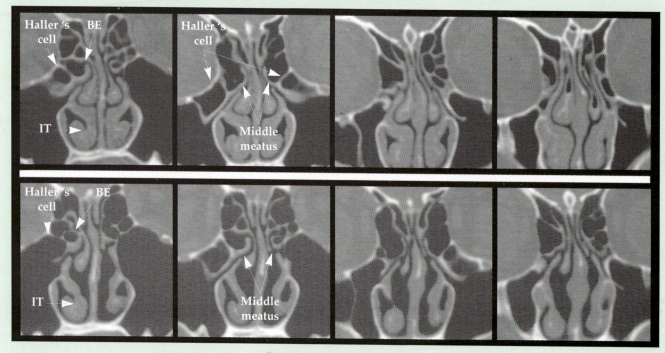

Postoperative CT scan

Paradoxical Concha

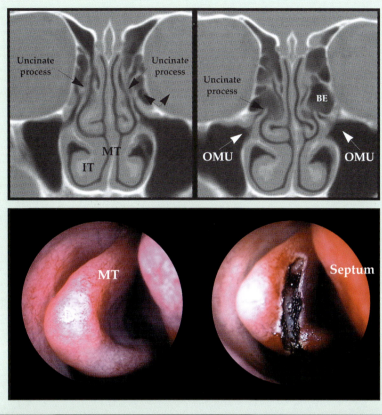

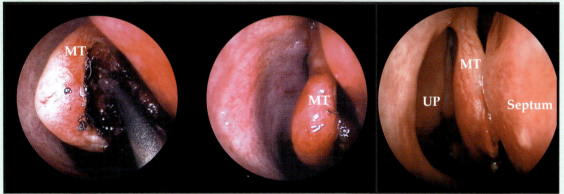

A paradoxical middle turbinate may produce ostiomeatal unit obstruction, as illustrated here. In this case the right nasal cavity is involved. The portion of the paradoxical turbinate that compresses the lateral wall is resected and the turbinate is sculptured so that the ostiomeatal unit remains ventilated.

Sculpturing of the middle turbinate is performed to achieve a clear, unobstructed view of the ostiomeatal unit. This also avoids medial fracturing of the middle turbinate.

Fracture of the middle turbinate invites problems during surgery as well as during the healing period. During surgery a fractured middle turbinate flip-flops, with the movements of the endoscope further traumatizing it. Apart from bleeding, one may end up losing the entire middle turbinate. Occasionally the anterior lamina of the middle turbinate is in direct continuity with the cribriform plate. Blunt fracture of the middle turbinate will lead to fracture of the cribriform plate and thus increase the risk of cerebrospinal fluid rhinorrhea, tearing of the anterior ethmoid vessel and difficulty in postoperative care due to lateral wall adhesions.

Conchoplasty

In a large number of symptomatic cases, radiological examination reveals only a concha bullosa. No ethmoid cell or maxillary sinus disease is evident. Traditionally, even in such cases, surgeons resect part of the middle turbinate or the lateral wall. We believe this to be overkill. In such instances we recommend reconstruction of the middle meatus with conchoplasty. In the method that we use, an incision is first made on the mucosa of the concha bullosa. The underlying bone is then incised, thus opening the conchal cell. After the mucosa is lifted over the lateral lamella to form a flap, the lateral part of the bony lamella is partially excised and removed, leaving the mucosa intact. This causes the lateral part of the conchal cell to collapse, resulting in a reconstructed middle meatus.

The advantage of this method is that it maintains the integrity of the middle turbinate, resulting in:
1. Preservation of the mucosa with the least amount of scarring.
2. Maintenance of air resistance.
3. Negligible crusting (due to minimum raw surface).
4. Faster healing (two weeks).

Preoperative CT scan

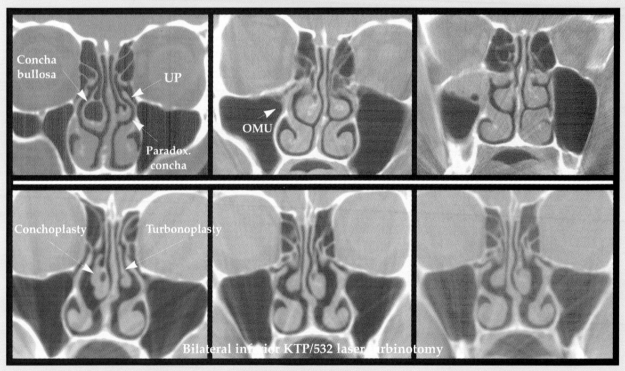

Postoperative CT scan

The above example illustrates the importance of minimally invasive surgical techniques.

A 42-year-old patient was suffering from recurring sinusitis. CT performed in 1994 revealed a right concha bullosa, a septum mildly deviated to the left and a left paradoxical middle turbinate. Conchoplasty and middle meatus reconstruction was advised. The patient moved to Texas and postponed the surgery. Symptoms persisted, and a repeat CT scan a year later revealed ostiomeatal disease. The patient returned for surgery. Right conchoplasty with middle meatus reconstruction, septoplasty and left middle turbinoplasty with middle meatal reconstruction was performed. Transcanine maxillary endoscopy revealed a normal inner maxillary ostium. Hence, the natural ostium was not disturbed. Two years postoperatively, the patient is still symptom free.

Conchoplasty

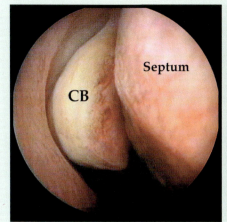

Right concha bullosa.

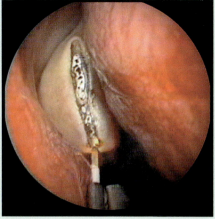

Incision with the KTP/532 laser in a near-contact method at 10 to 13 watts of power, continuous or pulse mode.

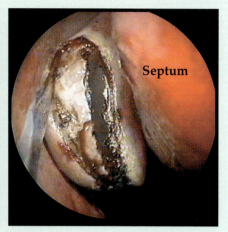

Elevation of the mucoperiosteal flap and its separation from the bony lamella.

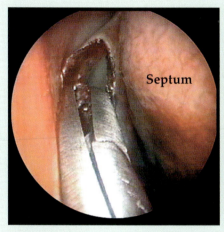

Partial resection of the lateral bony lamella with a Thru-Cut forceps.

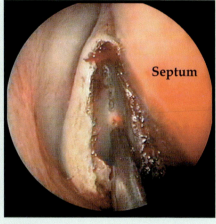

Incision on the posterior bony wall of the conchal cell.

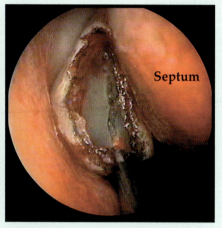

Incision continuing on the inferior wall in a near-contact mode.

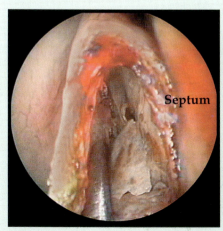

Fracturing the lateral half of the bony lamella.

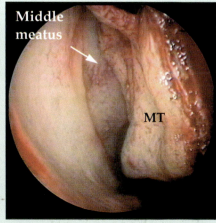

Draping of the mucoperiosteal flap and evaluating the middle meatus.

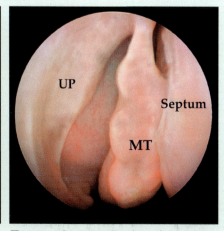

Two-week postoperative view with clear view of the middle meatus.

6

SURGICAL TECHNIQUES FOR OSTIOMEATAL UNIT OBSTRUCTION (GROUP II)

These patients have limited disease involving the ostiomeatal unit. They may present with unilateral or bilateral symptoms. On CT evaluation the disease is limited to the maxillary ostium. In our experience, minimal clouding in one or two ethmoid cells is nonsignificant. This is illustrated in the CT scan shown below.

Infundibulotomy with the Nick's triangle technique and reconstruction of the maxillary ostium is precision surgery. It requires accurate knowledge of the ostiomeatal anatomy. Experience in endoscopic cadaver dissection is essential. Refer to pages 38 through 41. The following case illustrates this technique.

A 50-year-old physician presented with a five-year history of recurring bilateral facial pressure, pain, postnasal drip and severe nasal obstruction. She had been treated with multiple courses of antibiotics, inhalant steroids, and anti-allergic medications. The patient was advised by another otolaryngologist to undergo endoscopic functional sinus surgery with ethmoidectomy and maxillary sinusotomy. Instead she underwent the minimally invasive surgical technique, as shown here, with complete resolution of all her symptoms. This is an excellent example of the tenet that aggressive surgery is not always necessary.

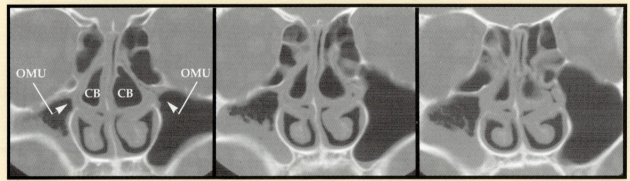

Her most recent CT scan revealed bilateral concha bullosa and bilateral ostiomeatal obstruction. Ethmoid cells were mostly normal except for mild clouding. The scan showed little change from the scan taken two years earlier.

Middle Meatal Antrostomy and Maxillary Ostium Reconstruction

Initially, an inferior third uncinectomy is performed to define the infundibulum and to reconstruct the ostium. Further resection of the middle third of the uncinate process may be necessary if the ostium is not found at this site. In our experience, we have not come across the natural ostium behind the upper third of the uncinate process.

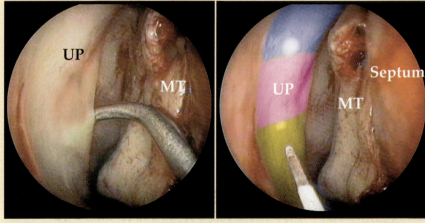

Define the entire extent of the uncinate process. Divide the uncinate process into three equal parts by imaginary lines.

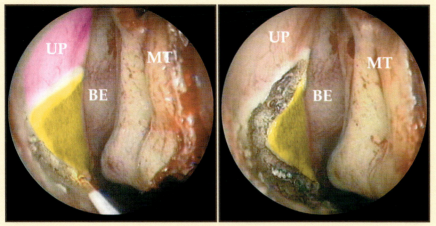

Use a laser incision to excise the mucosa down to the bony uncinate plate at the junction of the inferior third with the middle third of the uncinate process.

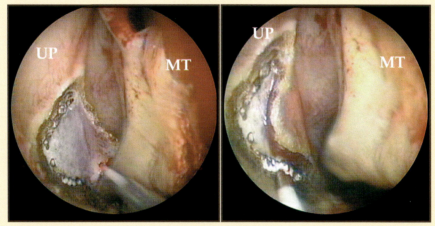

Incise the bony uncinate plate, keeping the laser in contact mode at 10 to 12 watts of power.

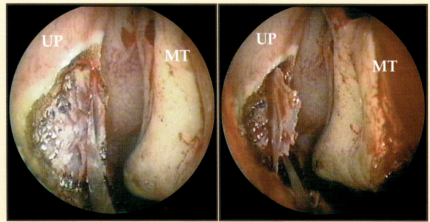

Remove the bony uncinate plate from the inferior third of the uncinate process. During this process, the posterior mucosa should be kept intact.

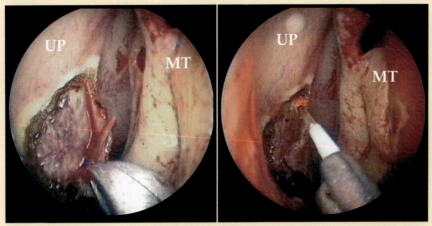

Use the KTP laser to incise the posterior mucosa without injuring the surrounding structures.

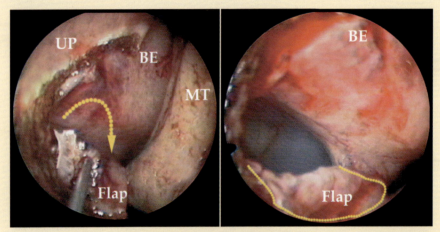

Reflect the mucoperiosteal flap medially and inferiorly, thus exposing the infundibulum. Inspect the maxillary sinus ostium.

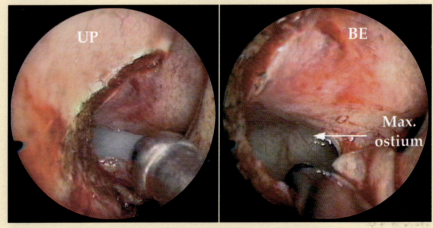

Remove mucopus and inspect the inner maxillary sinus.

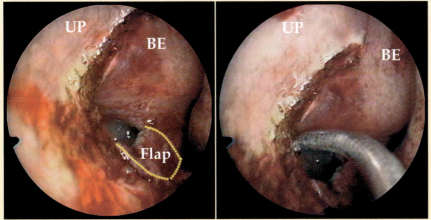

Use a ball probe to feel the upper extent of the infundibulum and the roof of the maxillary sinus. This maneuver ensures that the visible ostium is the only ostium in the infundibulum.

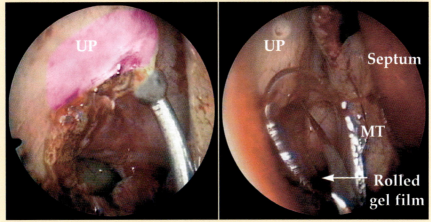

Move the ball probe behind the free and incised edges of the uncinate process to confirm its integrity.

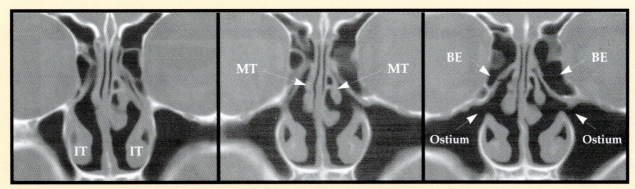

A six-month postoperative CT scan shows reconstructed bilateral ostiomeatal units, conchoplasty, septoplasty and inferior turbinotomy with preservation of natural ethmoid cells.

Maxillary Endoscopy

Indications

1. To evaluate the inner maxillary ostium when the presence of ostiomeatal unit disease is questionable.
2. Biopsy or excision of cysts, polyps, or tumors when the ostiomeatal unit is disease-free on CT scan.
3. In combination with middle meatus antrostomy to adequately resect the disease.

Relative Contraindications

Markedly hypoplastic maxillary sinus

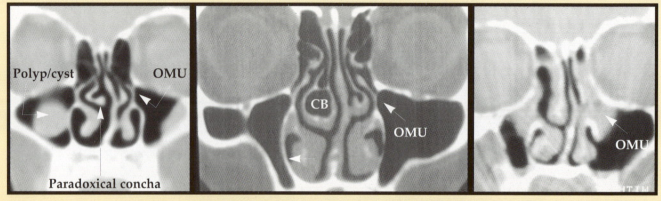

Isolated polyp or cyst with normal ostiomeatal unit on CT scan.

Inferiorly, a very narrow right maxillary sinus with lateral bowing of the medial maxillary wall makes it difficult to enter the sinus with a trocar without lacerating the medial wall. Hence, caution should be used when entering the sinus. In such a case the fenestration should be at a higher then normal level.

Bilateral ostiomeatal unit disease with hypoplastic right maxillary sinus.

Surgical Technique

The surgical procedure is performed under either local or general anesthesia. The patient is in a supine position with the head turned 45 degrees toward the surgeon for left-sided surgery and 45 degrees away from the surgeon for right-sided surgery. The following are important steps.

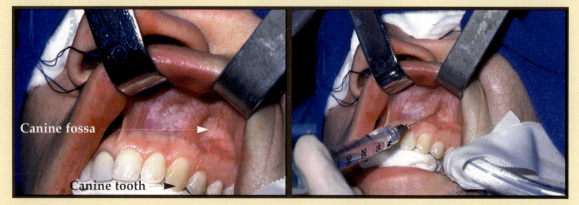

The canine fossa is the ideal site for perforating the anterior maxillary wall for evaluation of the maxillary sinus. The fossa is superior and lateral to the canine tooth. The canine fossa is injected with 1% Xylocaine with epinephrine 1:100,000 dilution.

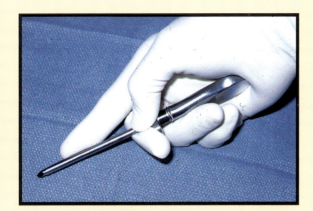

The infraorbital foramen is located approximately 6 to 8 mm below the infraorbital rim. Observe the position of the hands, the ideal site of the fenestration of the maxillary wall and the direction of the trocar with its cannula.

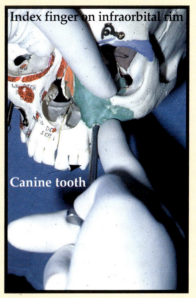

The method of holding the trocar with a sheath is important. The base of the trocar rests on the thenar surface of the right hand and the right index finger is extended along its length. This affords control of the amount of penetration by the trocar. The trocar is entered through the thinner part of the mucosa and submucosa of the gingivobuccal sulcus. It is directed approximately 45 degrees upward through the soft tissue. Once it reaches the bony wall, the direction is changed so that the trocar enters the bone perpendicular to the anterior maxillary wall. This ensures entry into the maxillary sinus.

If the trocar points medially or superiorly, it can injure the medial maxillary wall or the infraorbital plate respectively.

Left index finger remains on the infraorbital rim at the site of the infraorbital foramen. The left thumb rests on the anterior maxillary wall while the surgeon is performing the left maxillary fenestration. It rests on the maxillary zygomatic junction for fenestrating the right sinus. This maneuver retracts the upper lid and provides stability for a controlled fenestration of the anterior maxillary wall.

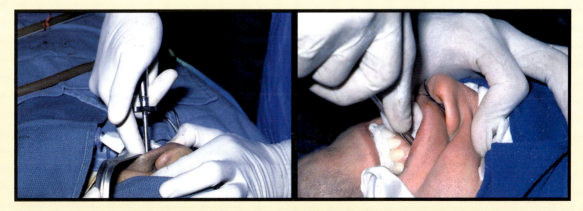

The trocar is advanced toward the sinus with a to-and-fro rotary movement. As mentioned before, the extended index finger prevents a sudden, forceful entry into the sinus, thus minimizing the risk of injuring the orbit and/or the posterior wall.

On entering the sinus, the cannula is advanced further. The trocar is removed only after the surgeon ensures that the cannula is in the sinus. Once the cannula is properly placed in the sinus, it is very important to stabilize the cannula. This should be done by the operating room nurse, who holds the cannula with both hands to prevent it from undue movement in the sinus. Excessive flopping of the cannula in the sinus can result in injury and bleeding of mucosal tissue, and injury to the infraorbital wall. This is a common pitfall of maxillary sinuscopy.

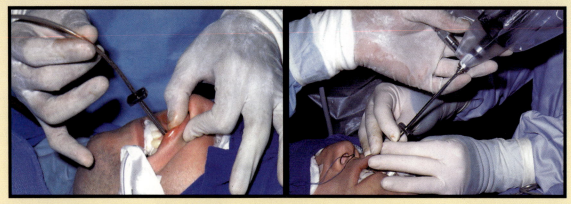

After the surgeon views the maxillary sinus with the endoscope, the sinus contents are aspirated and collected for sampling. The sinus is irrigated and then evaluated with 0-degree, 30-degree, and 70-degree endoscopes. In maxillary endoscopy, evaluation with a 70-degree endoscope is very important because in the majority of cases, the ostium floor and roof are not satisfactorily evaluated unless a 70-degree endoscope is used.

I am still not convinced that in the absence of definite ostiomeatal disease on CT scan, the cysts and polyps seen in the maxillary sinus have any causal relationship with the ostiomeatal unit. Hence, it is important to do a maxillary endoscopy and evaluate the inner maxillary ostium in all doubtful cases of ostiomeatal disease. The dye study helps in the evaluation of the mucociliary flow through the ostium. Diluted methylene blue is instilled in the maxillary sinus, excess is washed away, and the flow is observed. This, along with the condition of the inner maxillary mucosa, determines the need for ostiomeatal unit surgery.

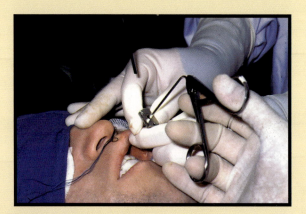

Techniques of biopsy and excision of polyps and cysts:
A 0-degree endoscope is used to view and approach the polyp, cyst, or the lesion. The cannula is used to tent the lesion and the endoscope is withdrawn. The biopsy forceps are then inserted and the lesion removed. This step is mostly a blind procedure. Tactile sensation and experience are important for adequate resection of such a lesion. A complete and thorough resection of such a lesion is generally not possible without a mini-modified Caldwell-Luc procedure, which we reserve for a second-stage procedure or for children with antrochoanal polyps with a normal ostiomeatal unit. The ostiomeatal unit can always be reconstructed as a second-stage procedure if needed.

In a modified mini-Caldwell-Luc procedure, the maxillary sinus is approached directly through the gingivobuccal sulcus incision. However, the resection of the tissue is limited, targeting resection of the cyst or polyp only. The healthy mucosa of the maxillary walls, and the ostiomeatal unit are left untouched. A nasoantral window is not created nor is the maxillary sinus packed. The entire procedure is carried out under endoscopic control.

This case shows isolated lesions in the right maxillary sinus with a normal ostiomeatal unit. The dye study shows a normal mucociliary flow in the inner maxillary ostium. Subtotal resection of the lesions was performed through the endoscope. Observe the dye flow study.

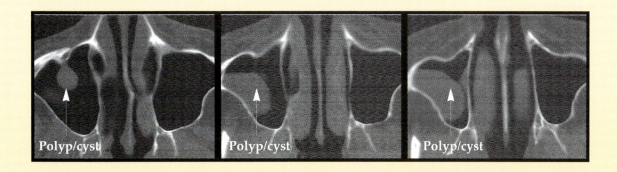
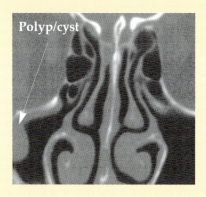
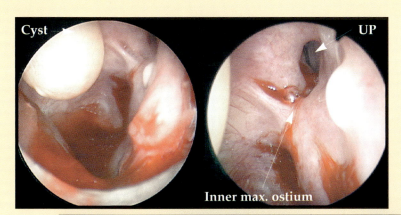
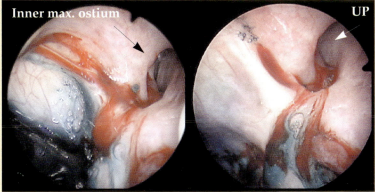
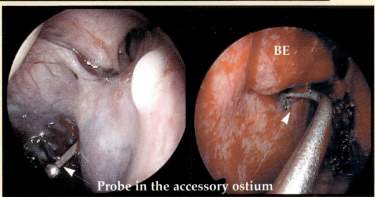
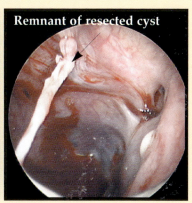

This second case was a challenge. There was a prolonged history of recurring right facial pain and congestion, all relieved temporarily with antibiotics. Nasal endoscopy revealed a normal-appearing middle meatus. However, the CT showed ostiomeatal unit disease. In addition, it revealed a tooth, protruding in the maxillary sinus. Canine fossa endoscopy was then done. This showed the protruding tooth which was covered with thickened mucosa. Tapping on the tooth with the endoscope did not elicit any pain. There was no tenderness on pressure. A diseased ostiomeatal unit with thickened mucosa was also seen. The dye study revealed an obstructed ostiomeatal unit with polyps. The challenge was whether to remove the tooth, reconstruct the ostiomeatal unit, or both. A less aggressive route was taken. The ostiomeatal unit was reconstructed and the tooth was left untouched. The patient improved markedly. If the symptoms had continued postoperatively, the tooth would have been removed in a second-stage surgery.

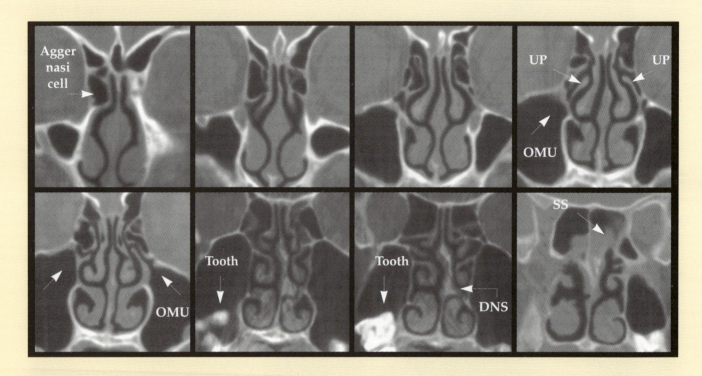

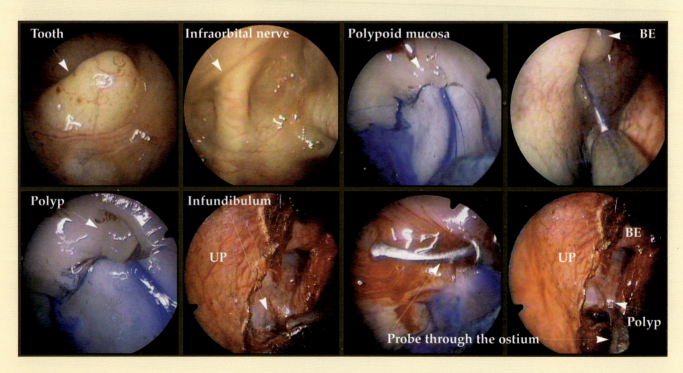

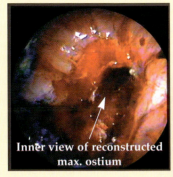
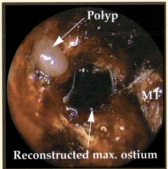
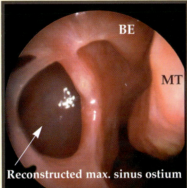
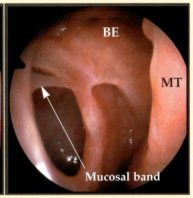

Six-month postoperative CT scan

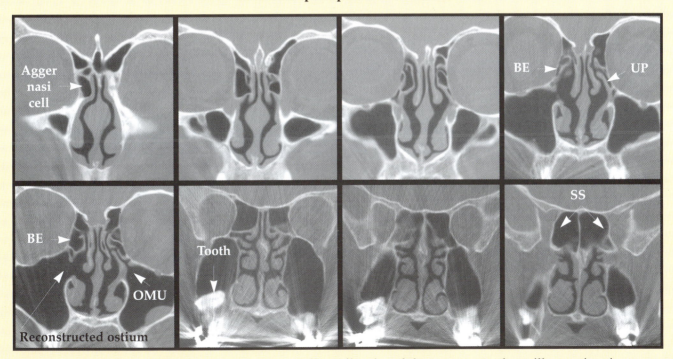

The septum is in the midline, all the sinuses are well ventilated, and the reconstructed maxillary ostium is patent. Note that preoperatively seen mucosal clouding in the sphenoid sinus has cleared up without operating on the sphenoid sinus.

A patient whose scans are shown below had a history of recurrent right facial pain relieved with antibiotics. Ostiomeatal unit disease is seen. Endoscopic evaluation of the middle meatus was unremarkable. However, chronic maxillary sinusitis with thick maxillary mucosa and a sluggish dye flow test with obstruction of the inner maxillary ostium necessitated limited surgery on the ostiomeatal unit with partial uncinectomy.

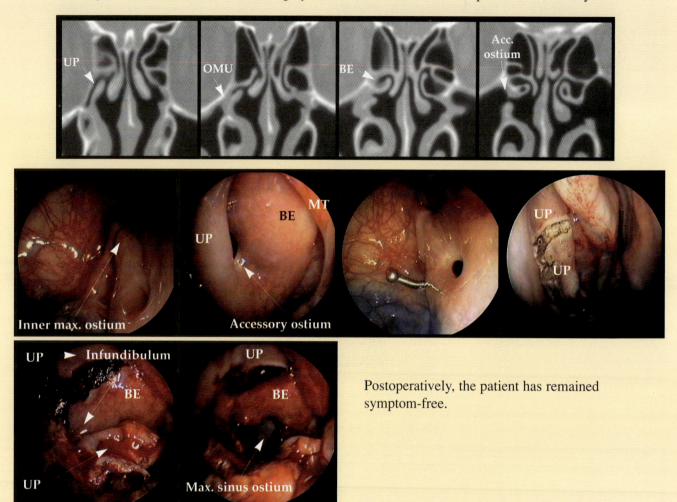

Postoperatively, the patient has remained symptom-free.

The case below shows an isolated cystic lesion attached to the infraorbital canal with a normal ostium. Endoscopic resection was performed.

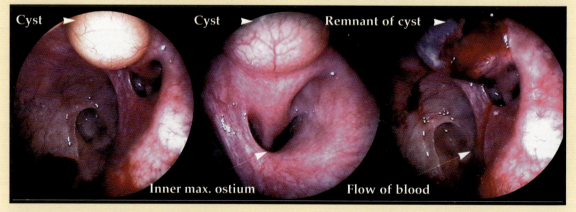

With a normal ostiomeatal unit and normal inner maxillary mucosa, the cysts and/or polyps are resected but the ostiomeatal unit is left undisturbed. Resection of the ostiomeatal unit in such conditions can itself lead to future maxillary sinusitis. Observe the flow of blood toward the natural ostium, indicating normal mucociliary activity.

Maxillary Ostium Reconstruction With the Microdebrider

The first generation of microdebriders was generally successful in resection of polyps and soft tissues. However, in bony ethmoidal septal resection, it was usually unsuccessful. The main problems were frequent clogging and insufficient power for resection. The newest microdebrider, the Straightshot Micro Resector System, has significant improvements including an excellent suction device, a lightweight handpiece and the ability to not only resect polyps but also to resect bony lamella. It rarely clogs during surgery and when it does, a disposable metal probe provided by the manufacturer aids in immediate removal of the clog.

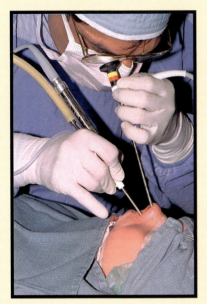

I have used the microdebrider for minimally invasive surgical techniques including polyp resections, limited ethmoidectomy, total ethmoidectomy, sphenoethmoidectomy, sphenoidotomy and frontal recess surgery. This impressive instrument also enables me to shave the ascending process of the maxilla, to unroof the agger cell, and expose the lacrimal sac. Hence, one instrument provides two actions, that of the microdebrider system and of an irrigating bur.

With the Toby backbiter, the microdebrider facilitates precise reconstruction of the maxillary ostium. Its use results in maximum mucosal preservation when compared with conventional techniques. The technique is easy to learn.

The following illustrates the use of the microdebrider for ostiomeatal unit reconstruction. Surgery is done under local or general anesthesia. The microdebrider should be held firmly and maintained in gentle contact with the tissue. It is kept parallel to the floor of the nose and is passed along the endoscope into the nasal cavity.

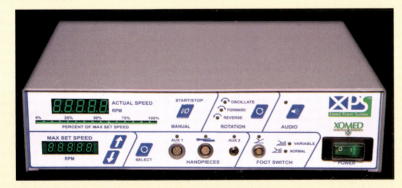

XPS Straightshot Micro Resector System by Xomed Surgical Products. The multi-function XPS Console allows operation of the Straightshot sinus handpiece, Powerforma high speed mastoid handpiece and Skeeter microdrill.

For uncinectomy, the microdebrider needs a rough surface to grasp. This is created by the reverse cutting Toby forceps. The forceps should be held as shown below.

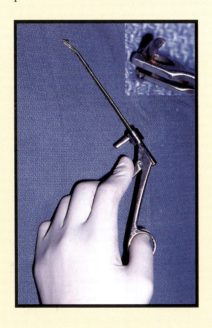

The following is a case study of a middle-aged man who presented with a prolonged history of recurring postnasal drip, feeling of bilateral nasal congestion, and mild facial pain relieved by courses of antibiotics. The CT scan below shows bilateral maxillary sinusitis with ostiomeatal unit disease. The anterior and posterior ethmoidal cells are relatively disease-free. In such cases the surgery is targeted only to the ostiomeatal unit. The ethmoidal cells are not resected. This minimally invasive approach is usually sufficient for cure in the majority of cases.

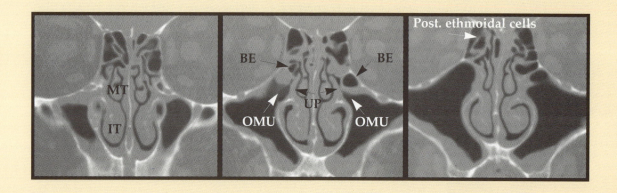

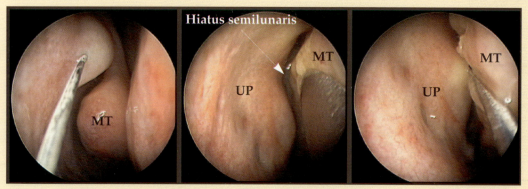

Local anesthesia is administrated. A 70-degree ball probe is used to evaluate the hiatus semilunaris and to define the condition of the uncinate process.

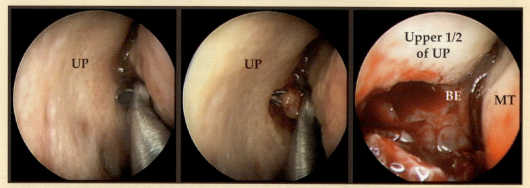

Insert the Toby microbackbiter and engage it behind the free edge of the uncinate process. Incise the uncinate process, separating the inferior half from the superior half by reverse dissection. The inferior part of the uncinate process is then reflected medially.

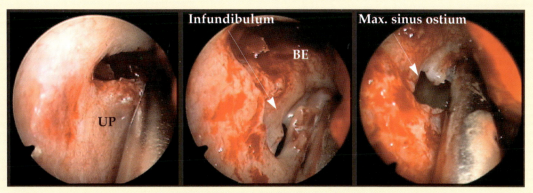

The microdebrider window is applied to the reflected edge of the uncinate process. The suction effect of the microdebrider grasps the tissue and the oscillating action debrides it. The debrided tissue, blood, and purulent material are evacuated by the suction to keep the field of vision clear. The inferior half of the uncinate process is resected. The infundibulum is exposed and evaluated.

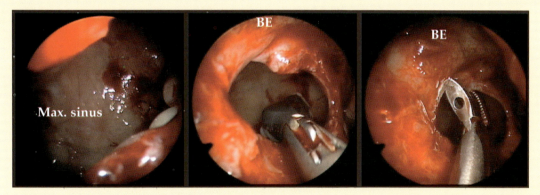

In this case, the ostium is enlarged at the expense of the posterior fontanelle. A polypoid lesion is resected from the floor with the giraffe forceps. A Thru-cut forceps is used to resect the diseased tissue, which is collected for histopathological examination.

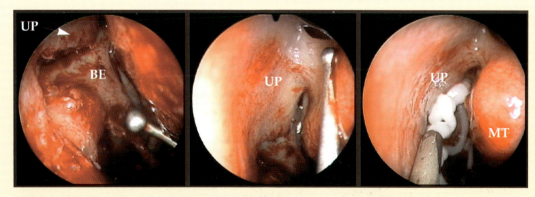

Water-soluble antibiotic ointment is applied and the procedure is completed. The upper half of the uncinate process is kept intact and the bulla resection is not performed since CT did not reveal any disease.

Two Ostia in the Infundibulum

The presence of two ostia in the infundibulum poses a challenge to the surgeon to identify the natural functional ostium. Canine fossa maxillary endoscopy with dye study helps in this identification. The following is such an example.

Precise infundibulotomy with the Nick's triangle technique using the KTP laser has been performed. The dry field achieved by the use of the laser has helped in visualizing and identifying the two ostia. With the given criteria, one would have expected the anteroinferior ostium to be the functioning one. However, it was the posterior ostium that was functional. Both ostia were connected with the KTP laser in the near-contact technique, and the inner mucosal flap was reflected downward. Connecting the two ostia with minimal trauma and without sacrificing the inner ostial mucosa should be the aim. This is done with the KTP laser in the near-contact mode. If as in this case the surgical aim is to connect both ostia, then identification of the functional ostium becomes a redundant step and the dye test is not necessary.

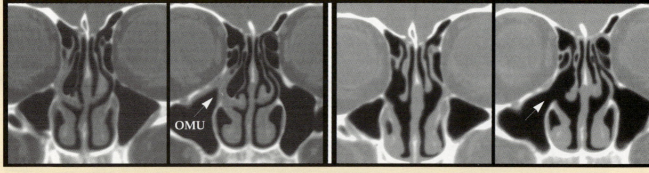

Preoperative CT scan

Right ostiomeatal disease, concha bullosa and left paradoxical middle concha.

Postoperative CT scan

Right middle meatal maxillary ostioplasty and bilateral middle turbinoplasty.

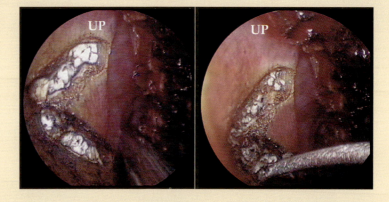

Infundibulotomy: the inferior third of the uncinate process is incised and reflected medially.

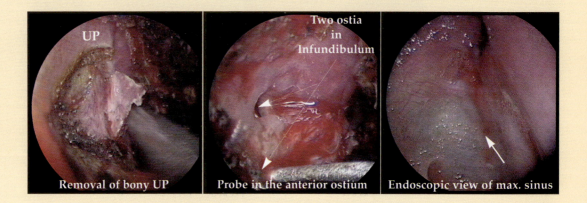

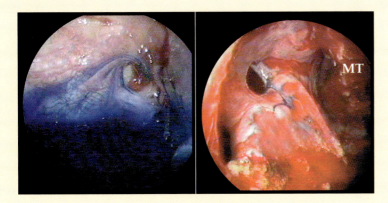

In the presence of two ostial openings, it is important to identify the functioning ostium. Transcanine maxillary endoscopy is performed, mucopus is removed and the maxillary sinus is partially filled with diluted methylene blue. The flow is then observed and the functional ostium is identified. In this case, it is located in the posterior part of the ethmoid infundibulum.

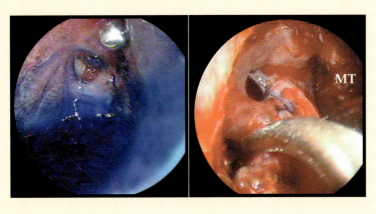

The ball probe is passed through the anterior ostium and is seen through the transcanine maxillary endoscopy. Observe the dye flow through the posterior ostium.

The bridge between the two ostia was vaporized with the KTP laser in a near-contact technique. The inner infundibular mucosa was reflected over the inferior turbinate.

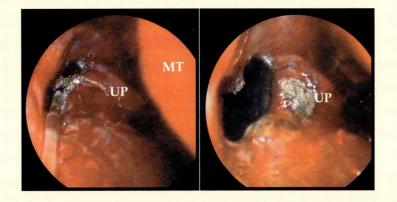

Two years postoperatively, the patient remains disease free.

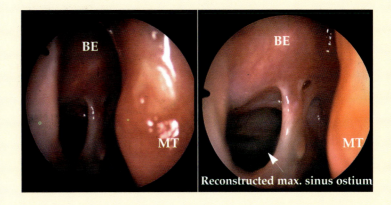

Serial Depiction of Surgical Procedure in the Management of Chronic Maxillary Sinusitis

A 43-year-old man was seen with recurring symptoms of facial pain, earache and nasal congestion confined to the left side. Several courses of antibiotics over the previous three years had afforded him short-lived relief. Endoscopy revealed a paradoxical concha and an inflammatory polyp at the upper uncinate process. The ostiomeatal unit was hard to evaluate without injectable anesthesia. Culture and sensitivity testing showed streptococcus sensitive to penicillin. The patient was treated with Amoxil, 500 mg three times a day for six weeks. Eight weeks later he was still symptomatic. The following scans are from a CT study done after a 21-day course of Cipro. The findings coincided with his symptoms of left facial pressure. Although the patient had absolutely no symptoms on the right side, CT revealed minimal mucosal swelling in the right maxillary sinus with ostiomeatal unit obstruction. The following surgical procedures were planned: (1) Reconstruction of the left maxillary sinus ostium with partial uncinectomy and nasoantral window. (2) Right middle meatus reconstruction and evaluation of the inner maxillary ostium through transcanine maxillary endoscopy with dye clearance study. If the ostium was found be obstructed, we would reconstruct the right maxillary sinus ostium with partial uncinectomy. (3) Bilateral middle turbinoplasty with middle meatus reconstruction. The surgical procedures which were performed are shown here.

During surgery, removal of the sticky, cheesy material from the left maxillary sinus was difficult. Hence, it became necessary to extend the nasoantral window and connect it with the natural reconstructed ostium. The inferior and middle turbinates were preserved. Right maxillary endoscopy showed a clear and normal inner maxillary ostium with normal dye flow, as seen here. The ostiomeatal unit was not violated.

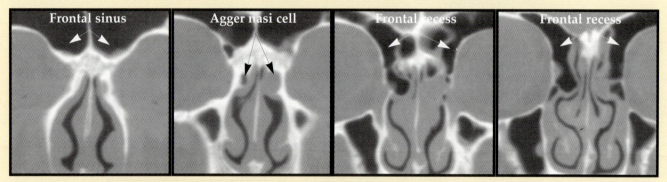

CT sections taken serially in an anteroposterior direction. These are presented in conjunction with the surgical steps. On the left side, note partial opacification of the agger cell with a clear frontal recess.

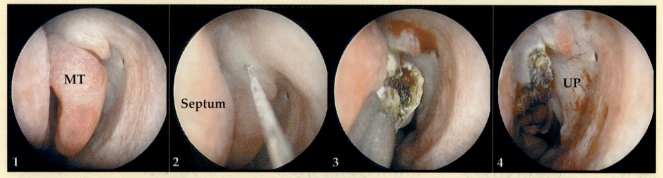

1. First endoscopic view of the left nasal cavity.
2. Local infiltration of 1% Xylocaine with epinephrine at the junction of the middle turbinate with the lateral wall.
3. A small segment of the anterolateral part of the middle turbinate is resected to visualize the entire uncinate process and middle meatus (minimal turbinotomy).
4. View after turbinotomy.

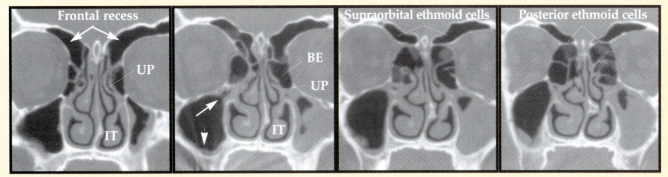

Bilateral middle meatus crowding with ostiomeatal unit obstruction. There is hypertrophy of the right middle and inferior turbinates with a mildly deviated nasal septum. Note that the patient is symptomatic only on the left side.

At this level the septal deviation is quite significant. Subtotal opacification of the left maxillary sinus and mucosal thickening on the right side are evident.

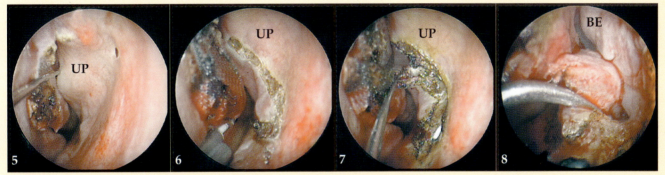

5. The uncinate plate is defined by wiggling it forward from its free edge by means of a 70-degree ball probe.

6. Incision on the inferior two-thirds of the uncinate plate.

7. Reflection of the inferior two-thirds of the uncinate plate.

8. The maxillary sinus ostium defined by using the ball probe. Care should be taken to prevent laceration of the inner ostial mucosa.

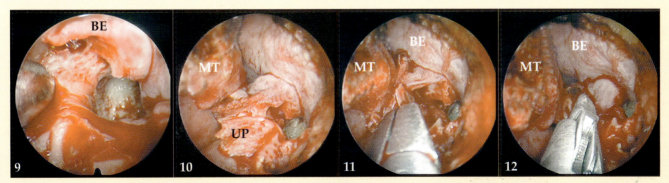

9 & 10. Reconstruction of the maxillary sinus ostium.

11. Submucosal removal of the uncinate plate bone.

12. Trimming of the uncinate plate flap.

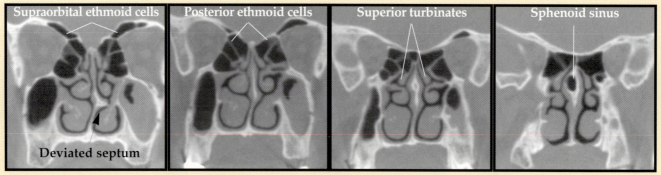

Hypertrophy of the right middle and inferior turbinates with a mildly deviated nasal septum.

In these sections, although the previously seen disease processes are evident in the maxillary sinus, the posterior ethmoid is disease free.

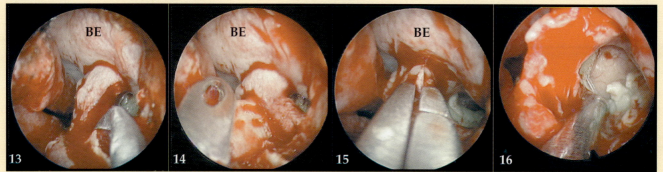

13. Use of a J-curette to perform inferior dissection and resection of part of the inferior turbinate bone.

14. Removal of a small part of the inferior turbinate bone.

15. Enlargement of the maxillary ostium at the expense of the posterior fontanelle.

16. Maxillary sinus antrum filled with cheesy material.

Inferior Meatal Antrostomy and Nasoantral Window

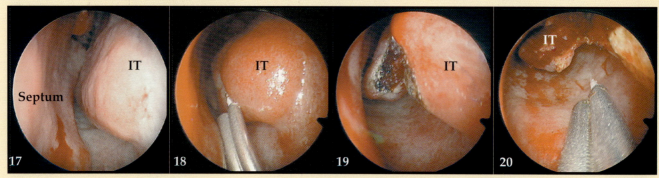

17. Left inferior turbinate.

18. Resection of a triangular part of the inferior turbinate at the site of the nasoantral window.

19. Site of the nasoantral window in the inferior meatus is 1.5 cm posterior to the anterior bulge of the inferior turbinate, flush with the floor of the nose.

20. Use of the KTP laser to create a nasoantral window.

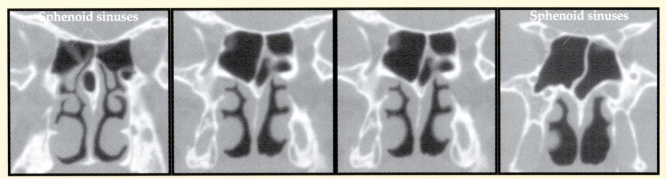

This section shows the posterior ethmoid merging into the sphenoid. It is of vital importance in posterior ethmoid disease.

These sections are through the sphenoid sinus. They help to identify the bony dehiscence of the lateral wall and the relationship of the optic nerve to it.

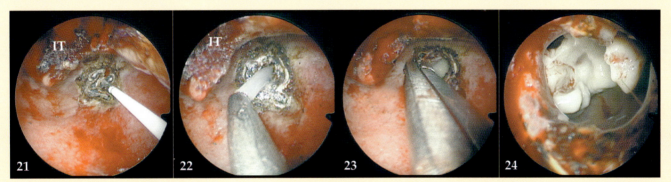

21. Vaporization of the bone to create a nasoantral window.

22. Removal of mucopus.

23. Enlargement of the nasoantral window posteriorly by resection of the bony wall close to the floor of the nose.

24. View of the maxillary antrum through the middle meatus.

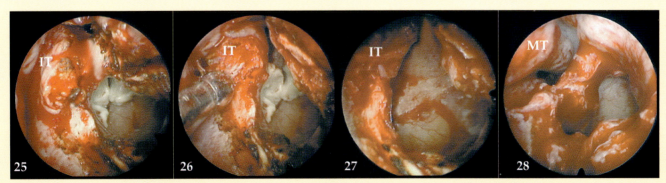

25. Nasoantral window being connected to the reconstructed natural ostium in the middle meatus by upward dissection.

26. Nasoantral window connected to the reconstructed natural ostium.

27. Disease removed from the maxillary sinus.

28. View of the maxillary sinus and ostial connection to the nasoantral window through the middle meatus.

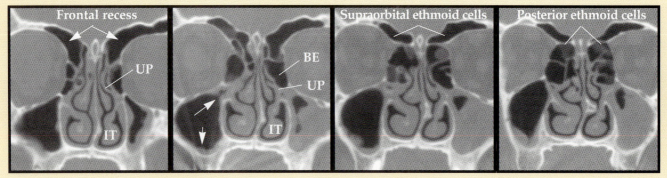

This patient was a challenge. Although CT evidence shows disease on both sides, the patient was symptomatic only on the left side. A decision was made to operate on the left side and evaluate the right.

Canine Fossa Maxillary Endoscopy

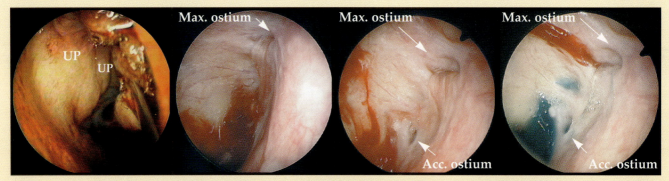

Right endoscopic view shows a normal, disease-free middle meatus.

Endoscopic dye study reveals a good flow and normal right inner maxillary ostium. Hence, the right ostiomeatal unit was not resected. The principle here is that when we see a normally functioning inner ostium, it is best to leave it alone, for man cannot reproduce what nature has given.

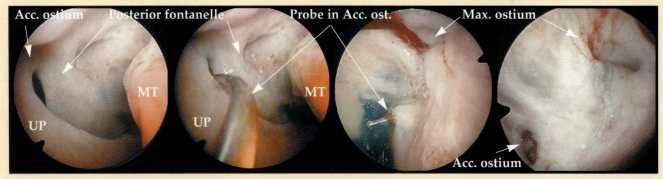

Right middle meatus view shows an ostium in the posterior fontanelle. In this instance, it is an accessory ostium. In approximately 11% of cases the ostium found at this location may be the only ostium. In these cases it is the functioning ostium. A careful dye study is the only way to differentiate between the functioning and the accessory ostia. Observe the normal flow of the dye and blood through the inner maxillary ostium. Although the dye collects near the accessory ostium, it does not enter it. It ascends toward the inner ostium.

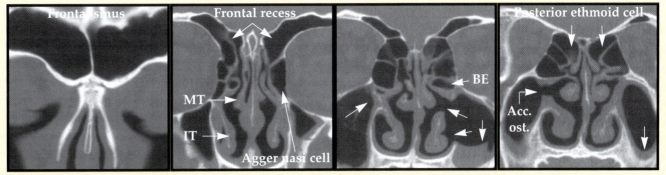

Six-month postoperative CT scan.
Observe the clear frontal sinus, midline septum, bilateral middle and inferior turbinoplasty and virtually untouched anterior ethmoid cellular anatomy. There is mucosal thickening in both maxillary sinuses.

The patient is completely symptom free. The right side again failed to show the ostiomeatal unit. However, there is significant improvement in the middle meatus as a result of turbinoplasty with middle meatus reconstruction.

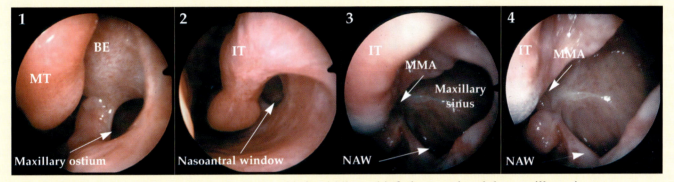

Three-month postoperative endoscopic views of left middle and inferior meati and the maxillary sinus.
1. Intact bulla, 1.5-cm reconstructed middle meatal maxillary ostium and the preserved middle turbinate.
2. Clear unobstructed inferior meatal nasoantral window. 3 & 4. Thickened, nonpurulent healed maxillary sinus mucosa. Nasoantral window connected to the reconstructed natural ostium.

Although the postoperative CT scan still shows some findings on the right side in the form of thickened mucosa in the maxillary sinus, the patient is symptom free six months postoperatively. The maxillary mucosal thickening seen on the left side in postoperative patients is considered normal when the patient is symptom free.

Nonintervention on the ostiomeatal unit on the right side and minimal ethmoid surgery on the left was enough to cure this patient. This again emphasizes the point that it is not necessary to be aggressive in surgical intervention. Excessive surgery, by violating the natural maxillary ostium on the right and destroying the normal ethmoid mucosa on the left, would have put the patient on the road to future disease. At this writing, the patient has remained symptom free and disease free for one year.

Note: Another way to perform a partial uncinectomy is with the use of the pediatric back-biter. The blade is inserted behind the free edge of the uncinate process and the dissection is carried forward. However, there are a few disadvantages to this approach:
1. The anatomy of the infundibulum and the uncinate plate is so varied that it is difficult to be precise in the dissection. Preservation of the inner ostial and infundibular mucosa becomes difficult, because the back-biting action is a blind procedure. There is not as much control on the mucosal resection, and the visualization is poor.
2. Bleeding always accompanies the maneuver, and this obscures the pathology in the ostial region and the ostium itself.

As opposed to this, in this instance, the KTP laser produces a much superior and more precise resection with preservation of infundibular and inner ostial mucosa.

7

ENDONASAL APPROACH TO THE FRONTAL SINUS (GROUPS III A & B)

Principles and Technique

The ostium and frontonasal duct exhibit such wide anatomical variation that approaching these structures endonasally is not always easy. However, if done in a systematic fashion, it is not too difficult either.

Important landmarks that should be identified are:

1. Anterior border of upper one-third of middle turbinate and its vertical lamella.
2. Ascending process of maxilla.
3. Anterior junction of middle turbinate with lateral wall.
4. Nasion—anteriorly.
5. Lacrimal sac—anteroinferiorly.
6. Anterior ethmoid artery posterosuperiorly.

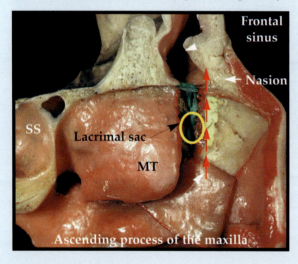

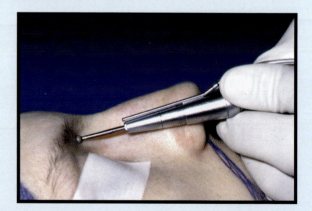

To adequately expose the frontal recess, shaving the ascending process of the maxilla with the power drill is crucial.

As shown here, in most cases following the ascending process of the maxilla while staying anterior to the anterior border of the middle turbinate will lead to the floor of the frontal sinus.

Exploration of the frontal sinus with drainage without identifying and addressing the frontal sinus ostium always results in a recurrence or failure of the surgery. Hence, identification of the frontal sinus ostium is of paramount importance.

In the following pages, the technique of frontal sinus surgery is illustrated step by step on a cadaver. This is followed by actual surgical cases.

1. Prior to surgery, review the CT scan taken in coronal and axial cuts. The sagittal reconstruction from a coronal acquisition is very helpful to understand the relationship of the agger nasi to the frontal recess.

2. In the first endoscopic view, identify the ascending process of the maxilla. Use the flat end of the freer instrument to feel the lateral nasal wall. It has a hard bony ridge, as shown here. Its posterior border corresponds to the anterior lacrimal crest.

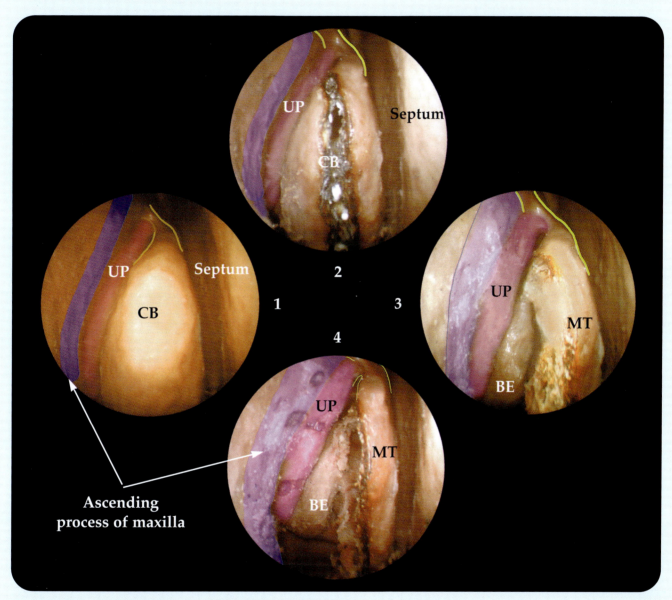

It is essential to have an unobstructed view of the recess between the middle turbinate and the septum to avoid injury to the cribriform plate.

3. The middle turbinate should be kept intact as much as possible. It is an excellent landmark. Staying strictly lateral to it protects the cribriform plate from injury. In cases of concha bullosa or a paradoxical or lateralized middle turbinate, a partial minimal middle turbinotomy is performed. In any case, the upper third of its lamella must be preserved. In over 55% of cases, the nasofrontal passage is located between the middle turbinate and the lateral wall under the attachment of the middle turbinate. The anterior border of the upper third of the middle turbinate is generally parallel to the ascending process of the maxilla. The floor of the frontal sinus is approached by following the ascending process superiorly while staying anterior

to the upper third of the middle turbinate. For the same reasons, one must make all efforts to preserve the integrity of the bony lamella of the upper third of the middle turbinate.

4. Visualize the entire uncinate process.

5. Divide the uncinate process into three equal parts. The upper third merges laterally over the lateral nasal wall covering the agger nasi cells. It attaches medially to the middle turbinate. Resect the uncinate process and delineate its upper attachment.

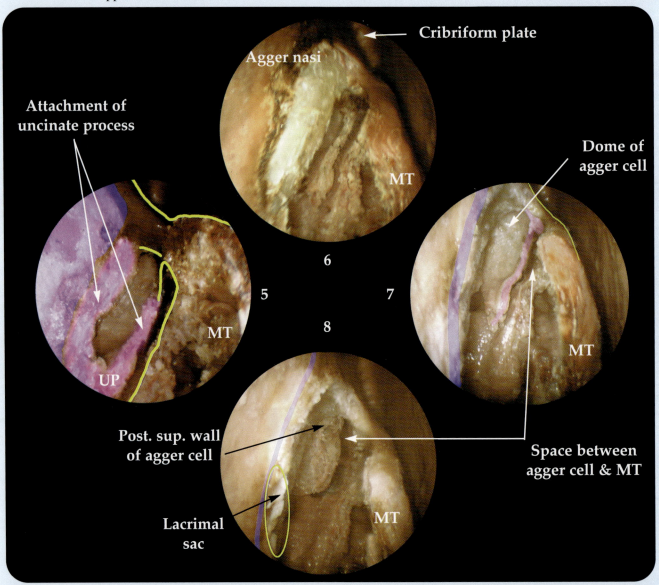

6. Resect the mucosa covering the ascending process of the maxilla in front of the lateral attachment of the middle turbinate.

7. Using a power drill with a diamond bur, shave the ascending process of the maxilla. Continue the incremental resection until the periosteum of the lacrimal sac is identified.

8. Now proceed upward along the ascending process of the maxilla to expose the entire anterior wall of the agger cell.

9. Identify the medial wall of the agger cell. Search for the space between the agger cell and the middle turbinate. Pass a curved ball probe or a small 90-degree angled curette behind the agger cell wall through this space. Take this wall down with an anteroinferior motion of the curette. This exposes the frontal recess.

10. Inspection of the frontal recess with a 70-degree endoscope reveals a medially located frontal sinus ostium. Note the lateral part of the dome of the agger cell. This should be removed to expose the entire frontal recess. Observe the upper attachments of the uncinate process. Medially it attaches to the middle turbinate and laterally to the lamina papyracea.

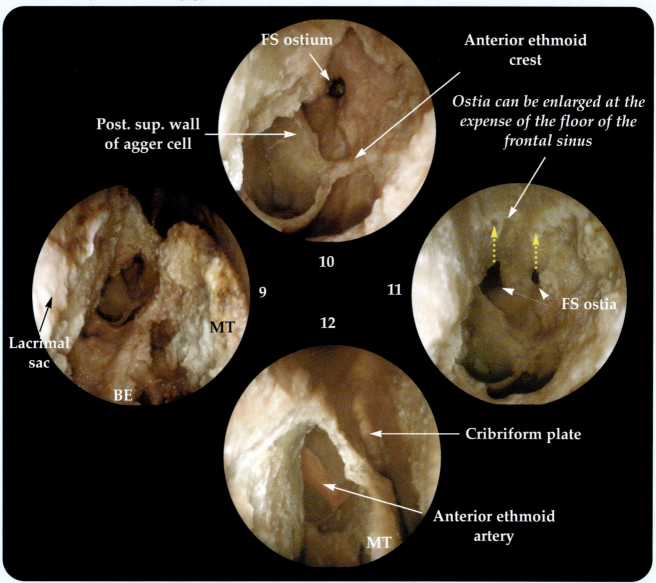

11. The entire frontal recess is now exposed, revealing a laterally placed second ostium. This cadaver had a bipartite right frontal sinus.

12. Posterior to the ostium a firm bony ridge is seen and felt. It is the anterior ethmoid crest. Generally, the anterior ethmoid artery is located 4 to 5 mm posterior to this ridge. Injury to this ridge should be avoided to prevent hemorrhage, intracranial mischief and postoperative scarring.

Frontoethmoid Disease (Group III A)
Recurring sinusitis with CT evidence of disease in one or two sinuses
(clear or partial frontal sinus opacity)

CT evidence of an air bubble or air-fluid level with partial opacification of the frontal sinus is a strong indication of patency somewhere in the nasofrontal pathway. These cases should be handled with extreme care. Relief is usually obtained by an anterior ethmoidectomy and clearing the disease from the frontal recess. Reconstruction of the frontal ostium is usually not required. Overaggressive mucosal resection invariably results in complete opacification of the frontal sinus. The surgical technique is described below.

A 38-year-old man had unilateral symptoms of facial pain, mucopurulent discharge and nasal congestion recurring several times a year. CT scan following optimum antibiotic therapy showed left frontal sinusitis with an air bubble, left maxillary sinusitis with ostiomeatal unit obstruction, a lateralized plastered turbinate without deviation of the nasal septum and hypertrophic turbinates. The ostiomeatal unit on the right side was not clearly visualized on CT, and a small focus of clouding of the ethmoid cell was considered insignificant.

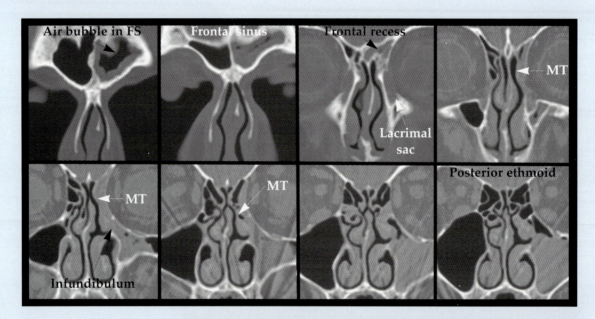

This severely lateralized and plastered middle turbinate was partially resected by KTP laser at 10 watts of power operating in the near-contact mode without fracturing the vertical lamella. The middle turbinate was resected with a sculpturing technique, so that there was maximum preservation of the mucosa and only the obstructing portion was resected.

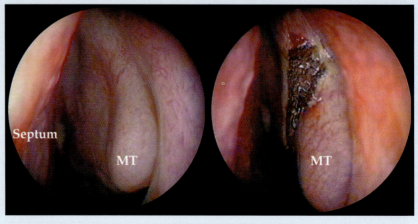

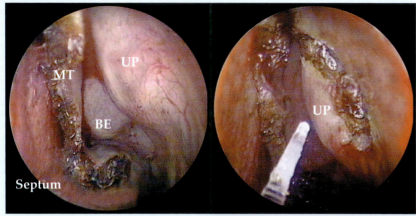

Subtotal resection of the uncinate plate is performed after delineating and preserving the upper attachment, which serves as a marker for the frontal recess.

The uncinate plate is reflected downward and medially, thus exposing the ethmoid infundibulum. Mucopurulent material is removed.

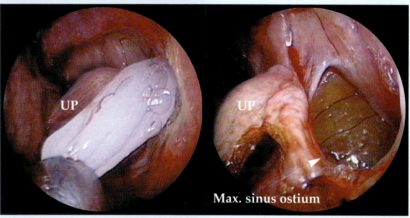

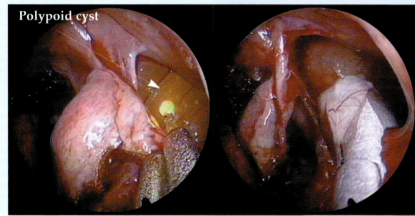

The enlarged ostium seen in this picture is a result of the expanding disease. If the disease can be reached and removed from this ostium, it is not necessary to enlarge it. This preserves the inner ostial mucosa and hastens the healing process.
The KTP laser was used to partially open a cystic polyp, and debulking was done with giraffe forceps.

The frontal recess is approached. In order to visualize it adequately, the bony arch formed by the ascending process of the maxilla with its anterior attachment to the middle turbinate must be partially resected. The first step is to identify this junction and remove the mucosa. Here, it is being done by the KTP laser with the near-contact technique, which provides excellent hemostasis.

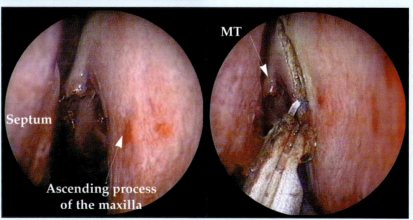

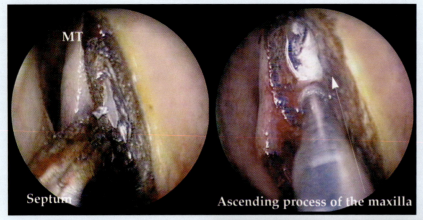

Incremental resection of the ascending process of the maxilla is performed with a diamond bur with continuous irrigation until the orbital periosteum is identified.

The upper attachment of the uncinate plate is followed superiorly and separated from its attachment to the middle turbinate. It is then resected downward.

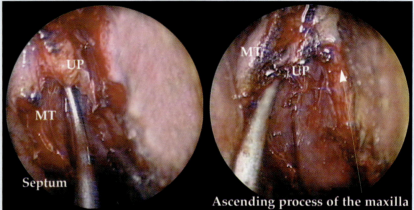

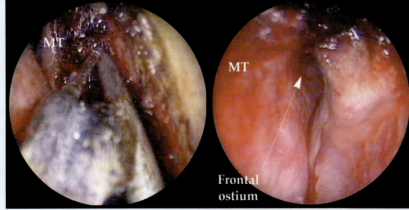

The frontal recess is identified behind the posterosuperior part of the uncinate plate. In the majority of cases, as here, the uncinate process harbors small ethmoid cells called infundibular cells. These cells are resected by placing the angled curette behind the posterosuperior part of the uncinate plate and making gentle downward movements.

After the frontal ostium was identified, the sinus was irrigated. Though not always necessary, here a 4-mm silicon tube was placed in the frontal sinus and sutured to the septum. It was done here because of the lateralized turbinate. The cannula is generally removed between three and eight weeks postoperatively, once the healing is completely satisfactory.

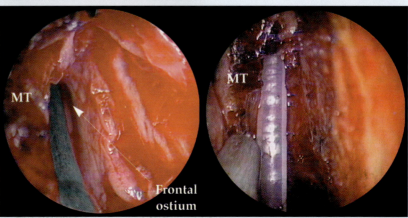

The four-month postoperative CT scan revealed a disease-free state. Right middle turbinoplasty and inferior laser turbinotomy were performed to improve the airway and to reduce crowding of the middle meatus.

Maximum preservation of the mucosa and the middle turbinate, clear identification of landmarks with excellent hemostasis with the KTP laser, and the use of integrated tools are the key ingredients of such a successful surgery.

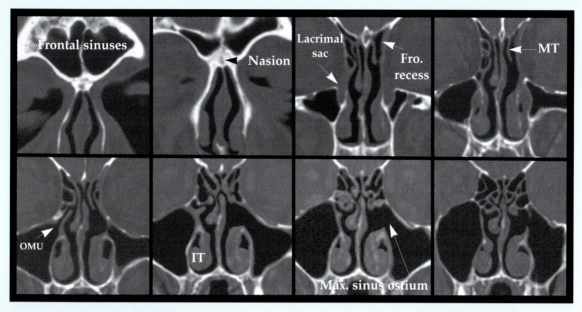

Postoperative images

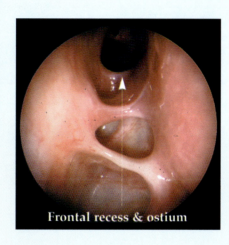

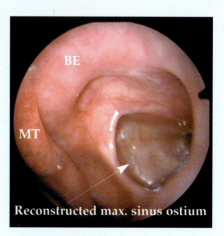

Revision Endonasal Frontal Sinus Surgery (Group III B)
Recurring sinusitis with CT evidence of disease in multiple sinuses
(complete frontal sinus opacity)

As previously discussed, if the frontal sinus shows evidence of air in association with other sinus disease, special care should be taken to avoid injury to the frontal recess. If there is injury to the frontal recess the result is disastrous, as seen in the following example.

This patient underwent an ethmoidectomy and resection of a mucocele by a combination of endoscopic and external approaches by an experienced endoscopic sinus surgeon. The disease recurred within six months postoperatively, worsened, and the patient was advised to undergo osteoplastic frontal sinus obliteration.

When I first evaluated this patient, the striking endoscopic findings were the complete absence of the anterior two-thirds of the middle turbinate and complete closure of the frontal recess region. CT evaluation revealed an intact posterior wall of the frontal sinus, dehiscent orbital walls of the frontal and ethmoid sinuses, and absence of the anterior two-thirds of the middle turbinate. The following is the CT scan prior to any surgical procedures. Compare this with the worsened postoperative CT scan on the opposite page.

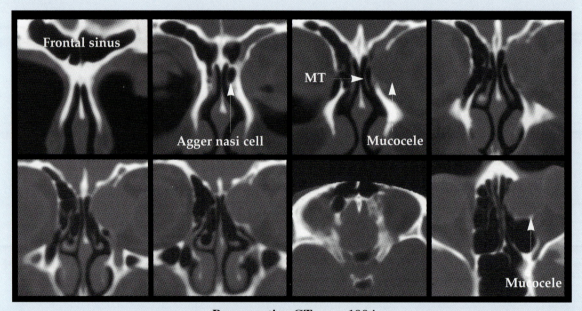

Preoperative CT scan 1994

Landmarks for Revision Sinus Surgery
In revision surgery, it is always a challenge to find proper landmarks. Following are the markers that I invariably find in revision cases in spite of total anterior resection of the middle turbinate:
1. Ascending process of the maxilla.
2. Remnant of the anterior junction of the middle turbinate with the lateral wall.
3. Lacrimal sac region.
4. Remnant of the vertical attachment of the middle turbinate to the skull base.
5. Maxillary sinus ostium.
6. Ridge of the junction of the lamina papyracea with the orbital floor.
7. Horizontal attachment of the middle turbinate to the lateral wall.
8. Fovea of the posterior ethmoid.
9. Sphenoethmoid recess with choana.

Postoperative CT scan 1995

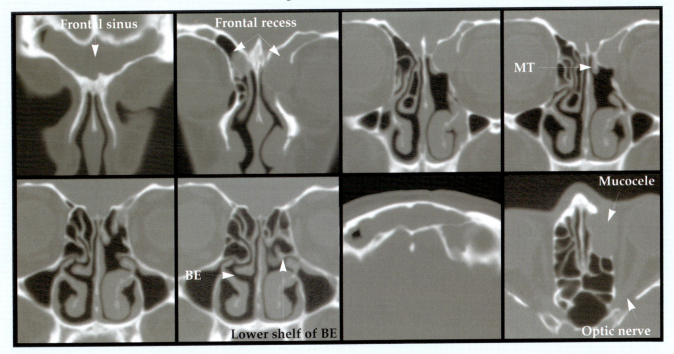

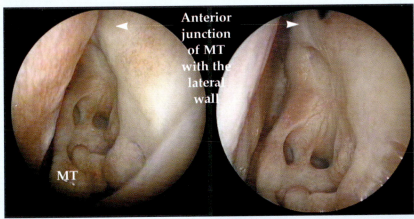

The surgical procedure begins by identifying the ascending process of the maxilla. Palpate the lateral wall of the nose, feel the firm bony ridge.

The mucosa over this ridge should be removed atraumatically.

A Fisch drill with a diamond bur is used to thin out the ascending process of the maxilla. Incremental resection of this process leads to identification of the lacrimal sac area. Gentle pressure on the medial canthus area produces bulging of the lacrimal sac. This is the anteroinferior limit of the frontal recess and serves as a good landmark.

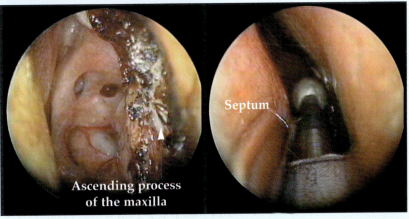

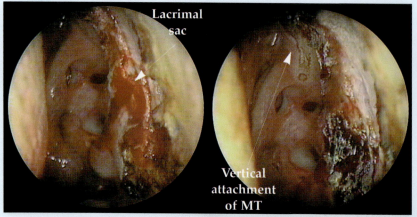

The next step is to identify the junction of the middle turbinate and the ascending process of the maxilla. This is the second landmark. The importance of this landmark is to stay lateral to it at all times during the surgery to avoid entering the cranial cavity.

The vertical attachment of the middle turbinate to the skull base is the third landmark. Dissection should be lateral to it because the cribriform plate lies medially.

Mucosal incisions here are placed with the KTP laser used in the contact mode at 7 watts of power.

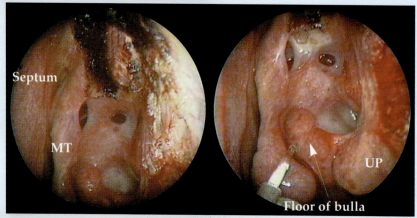

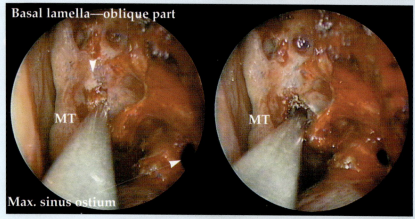

The next step is identification of the maxillary sinus ostium. Here, the inferior remnant of the uncinate plate was identified and reflected medially to expose the ethmoid infundibulum.

The posterior wall of the bulla was resected to expose the oblique part of the basal lamella.

Keeping the maxillary sinus ostium in view and hugging the inferior shelf of the bulla, the posterior ethmoid is entered through this part of the lamella.

Keeping the horizontal attachment of the middle turbinate intact helps ensure stability of the posterior half of the middle turbinate.

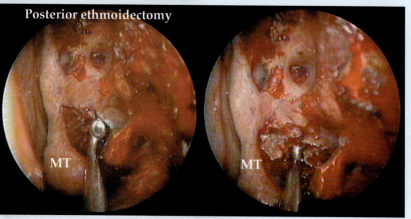

Part of the oblique lamella is resected to expose the posterior ethmoid fovea.

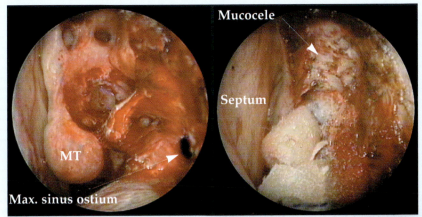

Now the anterior bulge is evident. The mucosa over this bulge is removed. This exposes the bony obstruction of the frontal recess. The bony part is resected with angled microcurettes, keeping the underlying mucocele intact.

Prior to incising the mucocele, all landmarks should be visible.

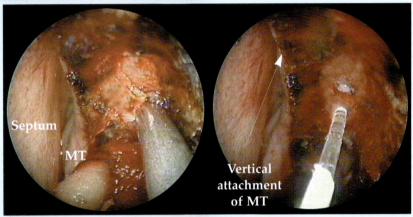

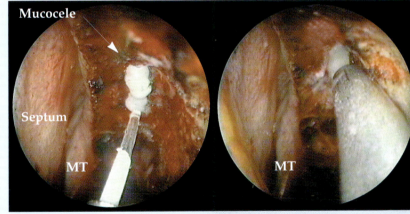

Needle aspiration may be performed prior to the incision. The incision is placed on the main bulge of the mucocele between the lamina papyracea and the remnant of the vertical lamella. Here, the KTP laser was used in the contact mode at 7 watts of power.

The mucocele was evacuated.

The incision was then extended posteriorly and anteriorly.

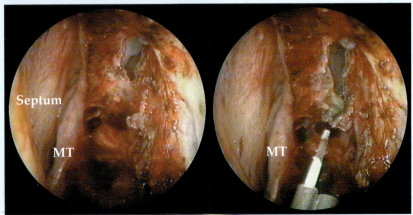

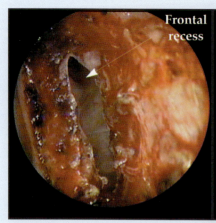
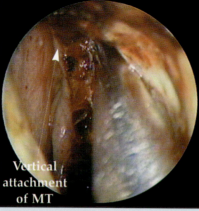

The frontal sinus was thoroughly irrigated. Here, the disease processes have created a large frontal sinus ostium that measures 8 mm in diameter.

There are two ways to confirm that the frontal sinus has been accessed. The first is to pass a curved suction cannula without resistance through the frontal recess. Place your finger at the columella against the cannula, remove the cannula, and apply it externally to see if it is properly placed.

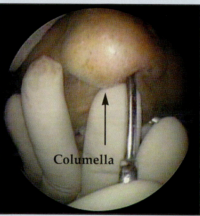
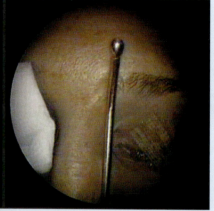

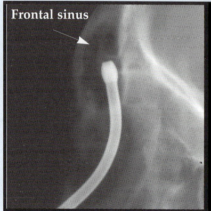
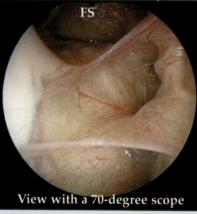

Lateral x-ray with the cannula in position confirms the position.

In order to make the anterior ethmoid cavity confluent with the posterior cavity, the septa between the cells were resected. Medially, septal resection was performed to the vertical attachment of the middle turbinate.

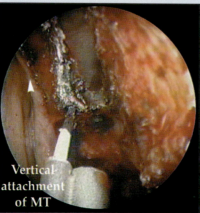
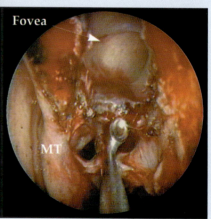

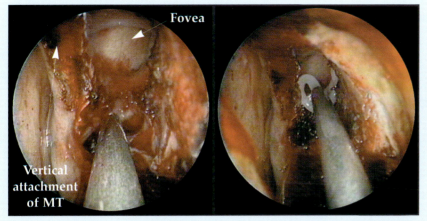

Surgery is concluded by application of water-soluble Bactroban ointment. A four-month postoperative CT scan and photographs revealed a disease-free state.

Four-month postoperative CT scan 1996

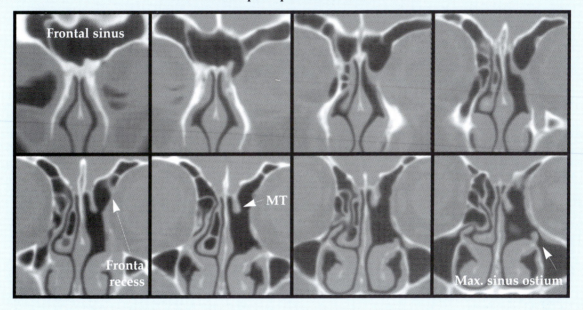

The aim was to marsupialize the mucocele intranasally with reconstruction of the frontal sinus ostium and to ensure its long-term patency. The surgical steps to successfully accomplish this are shown above.

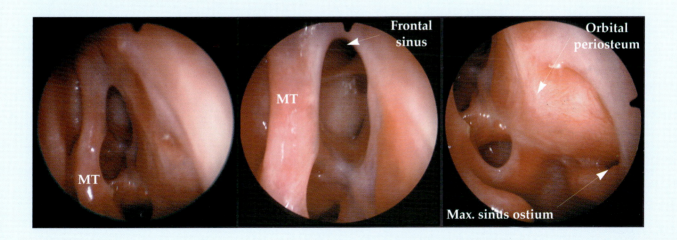

Pansinusitis with Polyposis (Group III B)
Recurring sinusitis with CT evidence of disease in all sinuses
(complete frontal sinus opacity)

Patients with CT evidence of complete opacification of the frontal sinus who do not respond to prolonged antibiotics and short-term oral steroids fall into a separate category and require special consideration.

The principles that I like to follow in these cases are:
1. Perform a thorough anteroposterior ethmoidectomy with preservation of important landmarks.
2. Address the maxillary and sphenoid sinuses next.
3. If the above steps are accomplished within a reasonable amount of surgical time (2-2½ hours) with minimal bleeding, and if visualization of the frontal recess area is satisfactory, then proceed as follows:
   a. Identify the frontal recess and expose the frontal ostium.
   b. Irrigate the frontal sinus and identify the pathology.
   c. If the frontal sinus is filled with mucopurulent discharge and the sinus ostium is of a reasonable size, leave it alone.
   d. If the frontal sinus is filled with a cheesy or fungal material and/or the mucosa is hypertrophic, additional ventilating space and manipulation can be accomplished by enlarging the ostium at the expense of the anterior floor.
   e. If the above is not possible due to poor visualization as a result of oozing, then do not take any chances. Wait, and do the procedure as a second-stage operation.
   f. If the frontal sinus is reached and its ostium is not addressed, the disease will continue.

What Professor Van Alyea wrote in 1945 is still true today:
> *"The health of a sinus is maintained only as long as it is lined with a functioning mucous membrane and equipped with adequate drainage facilities."*

During surgery it is imperative not to injure the mucoperiosteum over the junction of the posterior wall of the frontal sinuses with the fovea.

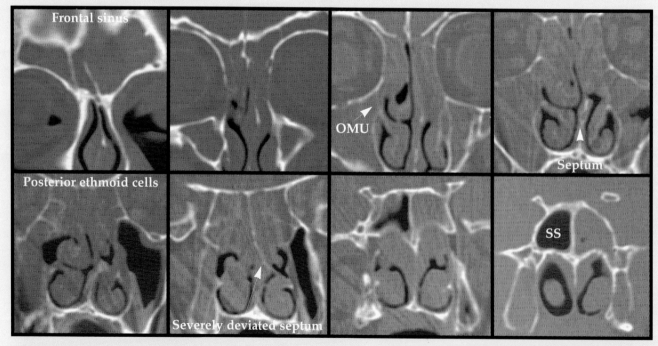

This case shows extensive pansinusitis with opacification of all sinuses seen on the preoperative CT scan. The septum is severely deviated on the left side. This needs to be corrected during surgery prior to the endoscopic approach to the sinuses.

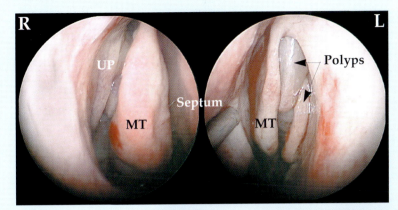

This endoscopic view is of the middle meatus after correction of the septum. When the middle meatus is clearly visualized without manipulation of the middle turbinate, the middle turbinate should not be disturbed surgically. Here, the left turbinate is very thin and delicate. Special care should be taken to avoid injuring it as this results in postoperative plastering and lateralization.

On the left side, the KTP laser is the primary instrument.

On the right side, the microdebrider is the primary instrument.

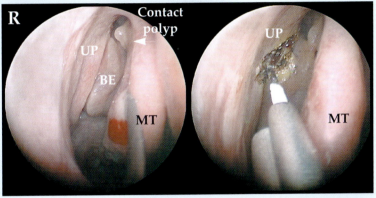

Use of Microdebrider

Here, the KTP laser is used to define Nick's triangle. In the absence of a laser, one may use a sickle knife or pediatric back-biter forceps with some restrictions. Refer to pages 38, 95 and 96.

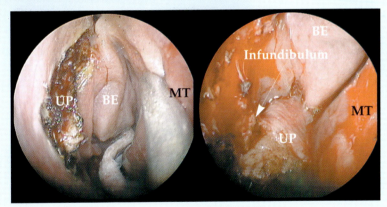

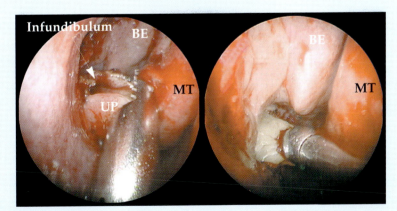

The microdebrider is used to debride and refine the incised uncinate plate. Gentle tugging with the microdebrider reflects the uncinate plate and exposes the ethmoid infundibulum. A curved suction cannula is used to remove the mucus and further define the maxillary ostium. The maxillary ostium can be reconstructed at the expense of the posterior fontanelle.

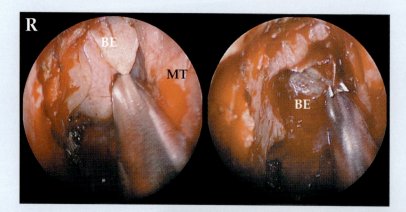

The bulla ethmoidalis is approached with the microdebrider and dissection is continued upward with debridement of the diseased mucosa and then through the bony lamella of the cells.

After disease has been cleared from the oblique lamella, perforate at its anteroinferior medial segment just above its junction with the horizontal basal lamella. This is the approach to the posterior ethmoid.

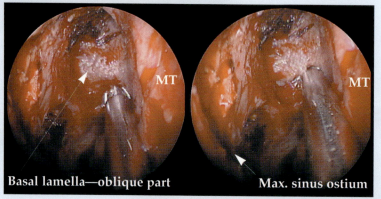

Using the 3.5-mm aggressive cutter in an oscillating mode, dissect the oblique lamella circumferentially. Avoid contact with the lateral and superior walls. The goal is to remove the disease and exteriorize the ethmoid while maintaining the integrity of the mucoperiosteum of the lamina papyracea and the fovea.

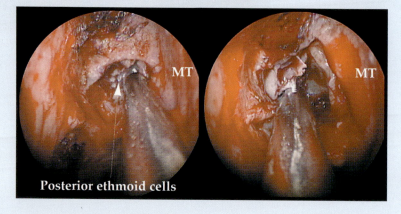

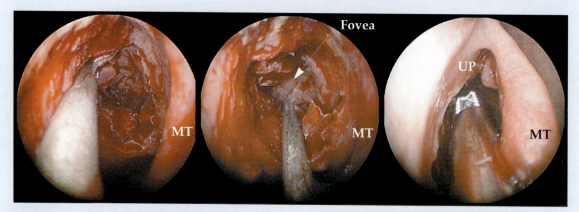

Identify the posterior ethmoid fovea before proceeding with the upward dissection. It is imperative to keep the fovea under constant visualization while resecting the disease. The posterior ethmoidectomy is now complete. Resect the anterosuperior remnant of the uncinate process.

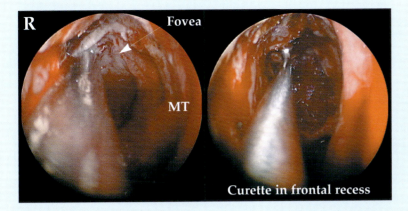

Continue the upward dissection to expose the agger cells. In majority of the cases the posterosuperior wall of the agger cell is not accessible to the microdebrider. To expose the frontal recess successfully, refer to pages 107 through 109.

Use of KTP/532 Laser

A polypectomy without causing avulsion, mucosal tears or disrupting the underlying anatomy is an art. The KTP laser is the instrument that is best suited to achieve this goal and especially to maintain the integrity of the underlying anatomy. This laser is an instrument which cuts, coagulates and vaporizes when the power setting is kept constant at 12 watts (12-15 watts, depending on the type of polyposis). When backed away slightly so that it is in near-contact mode, the effect is mostly vaporization. When moved into a totally noncontact mode, the effect is purely coagulation. A constant back-and-forth movement of the laser fiber tip from the tissue in a continuous lasing mode resects the polyps with some vaporization from superior to inferior extent. The tactile sensation from this movement gives you information as to where you are and a feeling of security that you are in the right place to outline the anatomical landmarks.

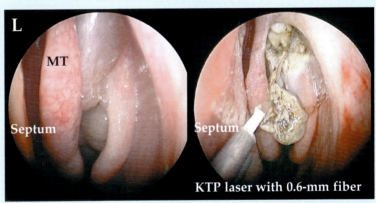

This near-contact sweeping technique is continued until the polyps are resected and the uncinate plate and the upper third of the middle turbinate are clearly visualized.

The next step is to do a subtotal uncinectomy, keeping its upper attachment intact as a landmark. The maxillary sinus ostium is reconstructed as previously described.

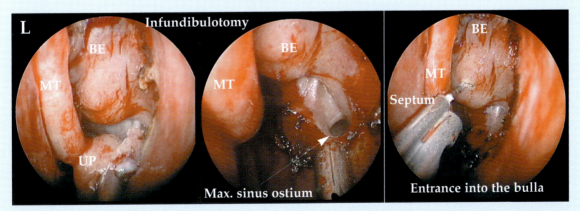

After maxillary sinus ostium reconstruction the ethmoid bulla is vaporized at its anteroinferior medial segment in a near-contact technique. The bullar wall is resected superiorly, with the landmarks (maxillary ostium and the upper third of the middle turbinate) always kept under visualization.

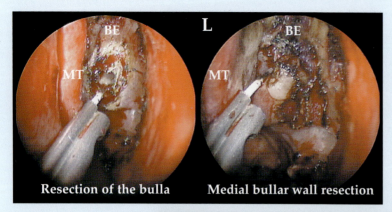

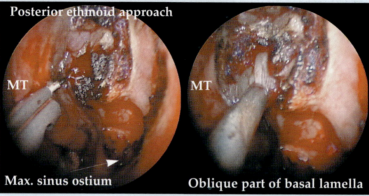

The KTP laser is used in the near-contact mode to vaporize the part of the oblique lamella just above its junction with the horizontal lamella. The posterior ethmoid sinus is then entered.

The cell structure is assessed with the dull ball probe prior to peeling off the polyps. Superior dissection is continued with the curette until the posterior fovea is clearly defined.

After the fovea is identified, the dissection is carried out in a posterior to anterior direction, with removal of hidden cells and septa. An angled microcurette is used for this. A dry field is achieved with the KTP laser, keeping the power settings between 5 and 7 watts. When a bleeder is observed, cottonoids soaked in oxymetazoline are first applied to it. Then the laser is used in a near-contact and defocused mode to coagulate the bleeder.

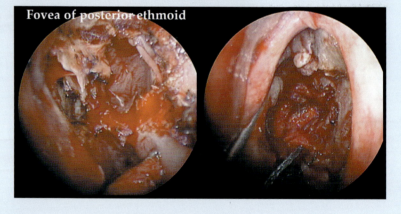

Two principles should be followed in treating a bleeder:

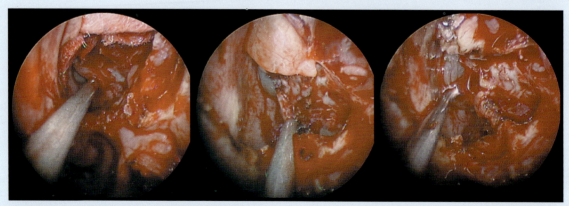

1. There should be clear visual control of the laser application. The bleeder should be clearly visible at all times. No blind application should be done.

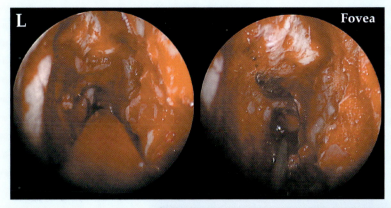

2. Be very specific in laser application. Unnecessary destruction of the surrounding mucosa is undesirable. If bleeding continues, apply compression. Remember that the laser seals vessels only up to 0.2 mm. Maximum mucosal preservation should be the goal, especially over the fovea, lamina papyracea and the lateral aspect of the middle turbinate.

The anterior sphenoid wall is lased, the sphenoidotomy is completed, and septa between the sphenoid and ethmoid are resected.

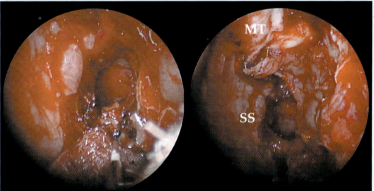

Conclusion

1. Always use the curved angle ball probe to assess the ethmoid cells close to the fovea and lamina papyracea before using the microdebrider or laser.

2. Important landmarks should be clearly visualized, as in this case, where hemostasis is quite satisfactory. The microdebrider and the KTP/532 laser are excellent instruments to clearly delineate the underlying anatomy.

3. The microdebrider is very good for the mucosa-sparing technique. It reduces tearing and unnecessary mucosal removal. It causes much less bleeding than the conventional technique. However, the KTP laser is as good as the microdebrider and in some cases such as turbinates and anatomical variants, even better for the mucosa-sparing technique.

4. The microdebrider uses mechanical force to resect the tissue. The KTP/532 laser uses photons to ablate the tissue. Not all polyps are the same. Some fibrotic and vascular polyps are difficult to remove without excessive bleeding. The newer microdebriders, in particular the XPS straightshot microresector system by Xomed surgical products, is a much better instrument than the conventional ones for polyps and sphenoethmoidectomy. The KTP/532 laser is better for vascular polyps.

The purpose is not so much to compare instruments as to demonstrate to all sinus surgeons how best to use whatever is available to them in the best possible way to achieve ideal results.

8
SPHENOID SINUS SURGERY (GROUPS III A & B)

Technique for Isolated Sphenoid Sinus Disease (Group III A)

It is important to understand and know a few anatomical facts before doing the sphenoidotomy. (Please refer to pages 48-51.) The sphenoid ostium is usually located at the level of the supreme turbinate. To reach this narrow and crowded area, resect the posterior two-thirds of the middle turbinate. Again, this is a very vascular area. Use of the KTP/532 laser maintains a dry field, which helps in recognizing the landmarks. To perform a direct sphenoidotomy, use the superior turbinate as a landmark and enter the anterior wall of the sphenoid sinus at its junction with the nasal septum. For an indirect sphenoidotomy, first do a posterior ethmoidectomy and then enter the sphenoid, as will be depicted. This route is taken when the ethmoid is diseased.

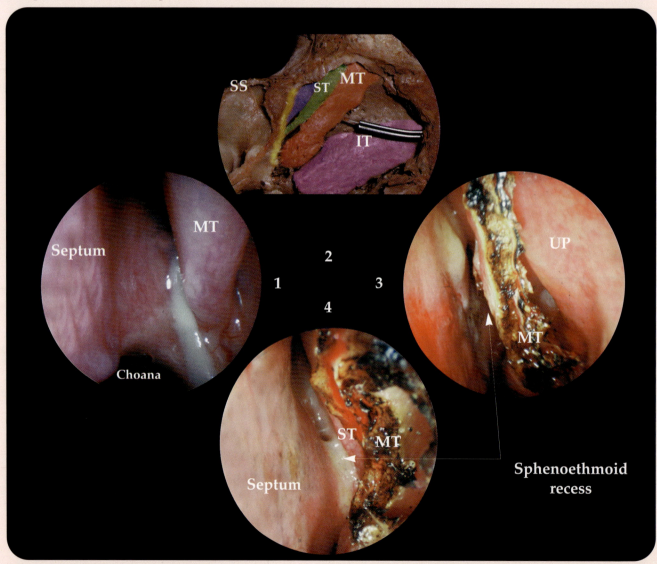

The first step is to define the partial resection line of the middle turbinate. The upper half of the middle turbinate is preserved. The oblique resection of the middle turbinate with resection of the bulk of the middle turbinate posteriorly allows definition of the narrow posterosuperior nasal space and improves accessibility. The KTP laser in a near-contact mode creates this partial middle turbinotomy with great precision in an absolutely dry field. This is essential for exploration of the sphenoethmoid recess.

126

The thickness of the bony walls of the sinus varies according to the degree of pneumatization. The inferior wall and the floor are generally the thickest. Hence it is difficult to perforate here. The ideal site to perforate the anterior wall of the sphenoid is 0.5 cm below the cribriform plate, where it is the thinnest—generally at the level of the supreme turbinate (in the absence of the supreme turbinate, just 2 mm above the level of the superior turbinate) at the junction of the anterior wall and the nasal septum. Attempts to perforate below this level may be difficult and may result in mucosal tearing. The septal branch of the sphenopalatine vessel crosses just above the level of the posterior end of the middle turbinate, and injury here can produce profuse and frightening bleeding. If the vessel is injured, first apply compression packing with Vaseline gauze. After 8 to 10 minutes of compression, slowly remove all packing. Identify the vessel and electrocauterize it with the help of suction cautery.

After anterior wall sphenoidotomy, use a curved curette to seek the boundaries. Enlarge the fenestration medially, laterally and superiorly, after feeling and identifying the recess behind the anterior wall with a ball probe. Small bites of the bone should be taken gradually with the sphenoid punch. With each step, a 90-degree ball probe or a curved curette should be used to feel the roof and the lateral wall. Connect the sphenoidotomy opening with the

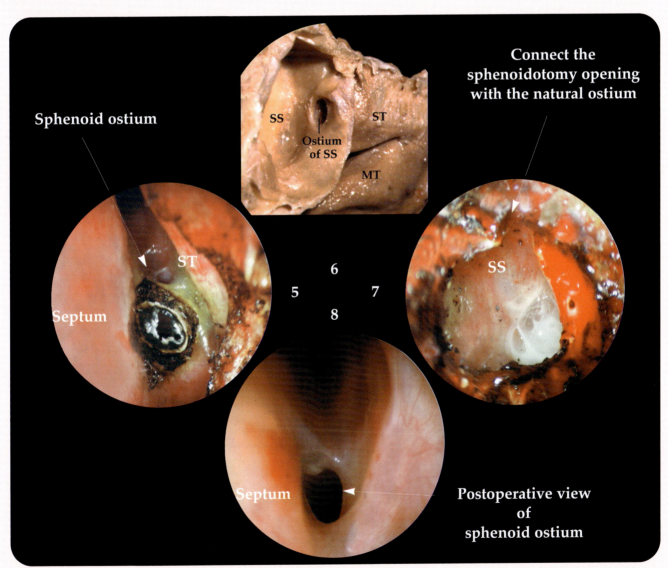

natural ostium of the sphenoid or the disease will recur. Intrasphenoid evaluation may show various types of septa and spurs. The septa can be partly bony and partly membranous, and may be complete or incomplete. Identify and study the septa on the CT scan before resecting with a Thru-Cut small-jaw forceps, taking small bites. Some of the septa end over the carotid or optic canal. If the carotid artery is lacerated while the surgeon takes down one such septum, death is inevitable. Blindness results from injury to the optic nerve.

Technique for Sphenoethmoidectomy (Group III B)

Penetrate the basal lamella to approach the posterior ethmoid with a pediatric straight forceps or a No.7 Frazier suction.
1. Localization in the axial (horizontal) plane between the middle turbinate and the lamina papyracea.
2. Localization in the coronal (superior to inferior) plane, just above the junction of the vertical and horizontal portions of the basal lamella.

Extensive dissection of the midportion of the ground lamella is to be avoided. At times, the form of the lamella is irregular and confusing. Either a well-developed retrobullar recess (sinus lateralis) or the bulla can indent the lamella and make it bulge deep into the posterior ethmoid, or a large posterior ethmoid cell can push the lamella anteriorly and disorient the surgeon. Second, overly enthusiastic removal of the basal lamella can destabilize the middle turbinate and result in a lateral drift with formation of adhesions to the lateral nasal wall.

The inferior point at which the vertical portion of the ground lamella of the middle turbinate joins the horizontal portion of the ground lamella is another reference area to help orient the surgeon for penetration into the posterior ethmoid. Perforation of the inferomedial aspect of the vertical ground lamella just above the point where it joins the horizontal portion is safe. This level gives good alignment of the endoscope and instruments for opening the posterior ethmoid and anterior sphenoid wall.

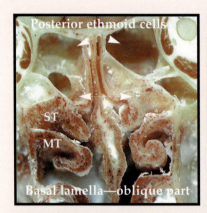
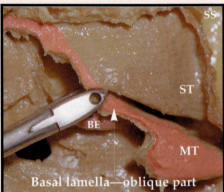
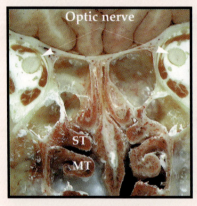
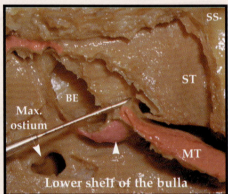
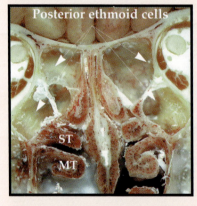
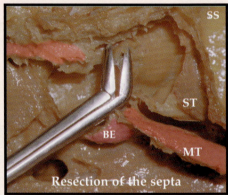
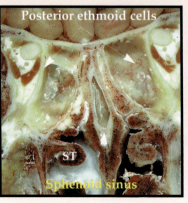
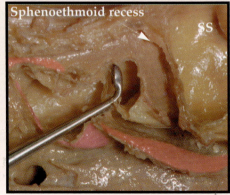

When visualized from its anterior aspect, the superior turbinate divides the anterior face of the sphenoid into a lateral two-thirds, a portion that is obscured by the ethmoid, and a medial third which can be visualized in the sphenoethmoid recess.

Never search for the anterior sphenoid wall in the deepest portion of the posterior ethmoid. There is a high risk of craniotomy or optic nerve injury. Enter the sphenoid ostium just superior to the point where the middle turbinate turns lateral to attach to the lateral nasal wall. Picture the anterior sphenoid wall as projecting into the posterior ethmoid-like nose cone of a rocket. Assess the shape of the sphenoid rostrum and penetrate the thin portion medially. A firm anterior sphenoid wall forces the instrument superiorly and laterally, causing inability to identify the sphenoid ostium. A C-arm is necessary if the ostium is not seen and the area of penetration is hard to access.

After penetration of the ground lamella and completion of the posterior ethmoidectomy, one must reorient for opening of the anterior sphenoid wall. Large posterior ethmoid cells can extend posterior and superior to the anterior sphenoid wall. When these cells are indented superolaterally by the optic nerve, they are called Onodi cells. In this circumstance, the configuration of the anterior sphenoid wall is usually sharply angled, like the prow of a ship, with a protrusion into the posterior ethmoid. Confusion as to the best angle and level of penetration can be significant. The best advice is to stay paramedial and just above the remnant of the junction of the vertical and horizontal portions of the basal lamella of the middle turbinate. This will help correctly direct the instruments with an inferior bias.

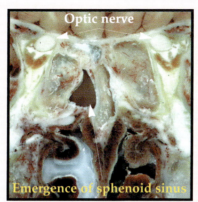
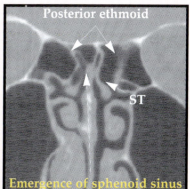
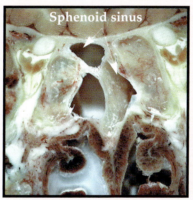
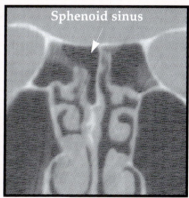
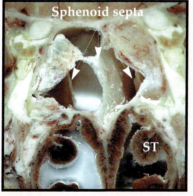
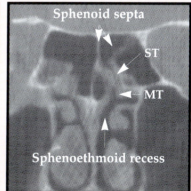
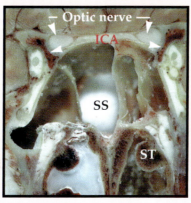
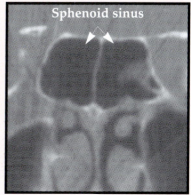

Posterior Ethmoidectomy and Sphenoidotomy (Group III B)
Recurring sinusitis with CT evidence of disease in one or two sinuses
(sphenoethmoid disease with clear frontal sinuses)

The sphenoid sinus drains into the sphenoethmoid recess. This space very often shares the drainage of the posterior ethmoid. When infection occurs in this area, usually both the sphenoid and the ethmoid sinuses are involved. This case depicts the sinus surgical procedure limited to the sphenoid and posterior ethmoid sinuses, leaving the anterior ethmoid sinus undisturbed.

A 50-year-old man presented with a prolonged history of occipital and diffuse headaches and right nasal congestion. This case was challenging as the patient was monocular, having lost his left eye as a result of trauma several years earlier. Endoscopic evaluation revealed an unremarkable right middle meatus and obliteration of the sphenoethmoid recess with edematous mucosa. Disease was found in the right sphenoethmoid, as seen on the CT scan. The following are pre- and postsurgical CT scans for a comparative study and to demonstrate an intact unviolated anterior ethmoid sinus and disease-free posterior ethmoid and sphenoid sinuses. Preoperatively it is imperative to obtain and study the axial and coronal CT sections through the posterior ethmoid and sphenoid sinuses to evaluate the condition of the lamina papyracea and the course of the optic nerve.

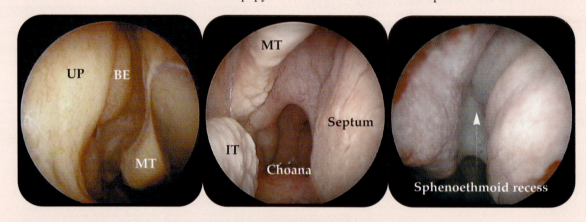

Preoperative axial CT sections

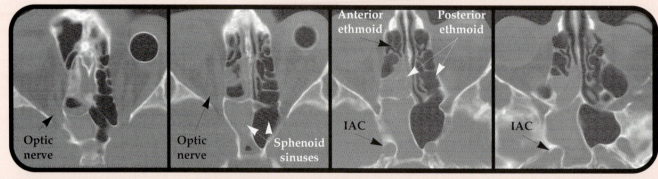

Four-month postoperative axial CT sections

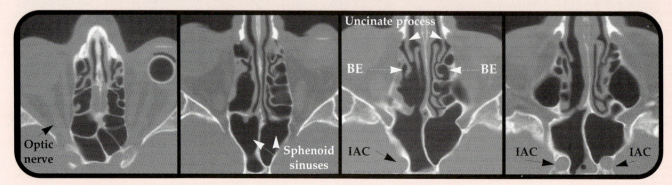

The axial view is important because it shows an artificial eye in the left orbit, good anteroposterior space of the sphenoid sinus, and no bony dehiscence, and the intrasphenoid septa do not terminate on the carotid canal.

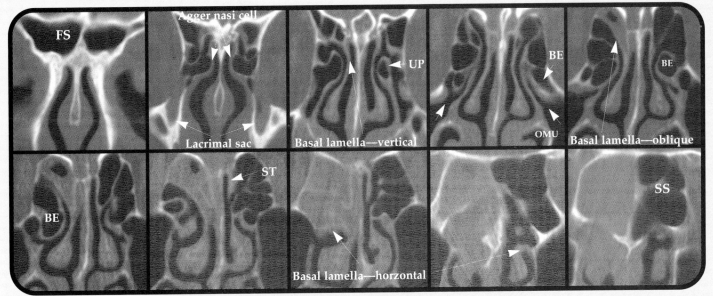

Preoperative CT scan

The CT scan revealed a clear anterior ethmoid complex. The disease process is limited to the posterior ethmoid with complete opacification of the sphenoid sinus.

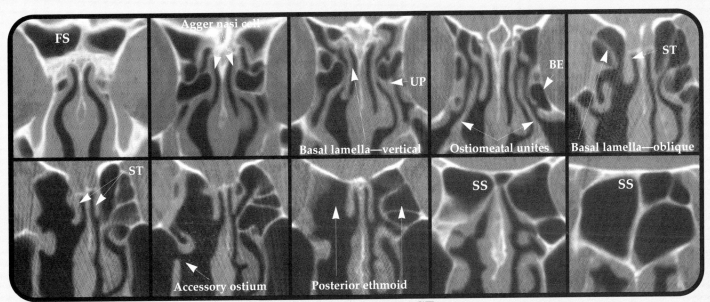

Four-month postoperative CT scan

The CT scan revealed an undisturbed anterior ethmoid complex. The disease seen previously in the posterior ethmoid and sphenoid sinuses has resolved, leaving a confluent cavity.

The patient underwent surgery after 10 days of oral antibiotics and steroids. The technique is as follows:

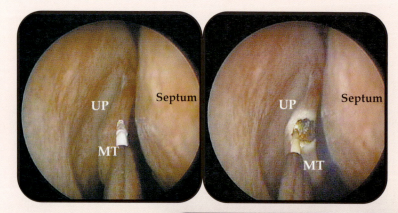

The first step is to define the partial resection of the middle turbinate. The upper half of the middle turbinate is preserved.

Oblique resection of the middle turbinate with resection of the bulk of the middle turbinate posteriorly enables the definition of the narrow posterosuperior nasal space and improves accessibility.

The KTP/532 laser is used in a near-contact mode to perform this partial middle turbinotomy with great precision in an absolutely dry field. This is essential for exploration of the sphenoethmoid recess.

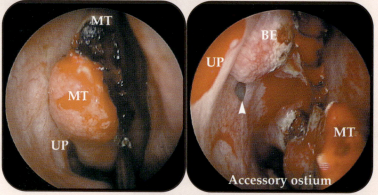

Part of the oblique lamella above its junction with the horizontal part is vaporized to expose the superior turbinate and the sphenoethmoid recess.

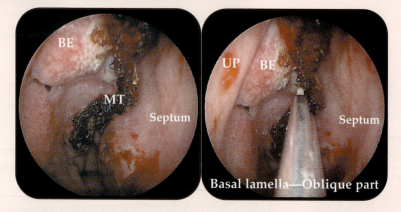

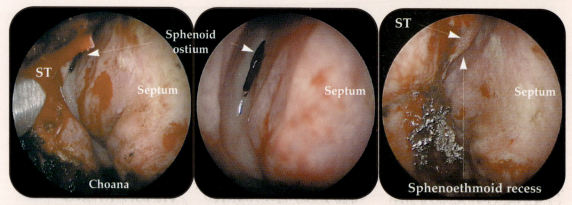

The sphenoid ostium is well visualized. The "scatter" property of the KTP laser helps to reduce mucosal edema and also helps achieve hemostasis.

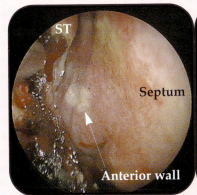 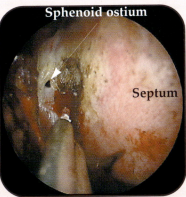

The junction of the anterior sphenoid wall with the nasal septum is vaporized in a near-contact mode after first achieving the coagulation effect on the mucosa. This site is below the sphenoid ostium. Tactile sensation plays a very important role here.

I feel the bone with the tip of the KTP laser fiber, then pull back to come in the near-contact position before vaporization. Several such spots are vaporized and the vaporized bone is removed with a Frazier suction.

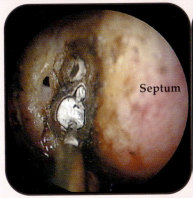 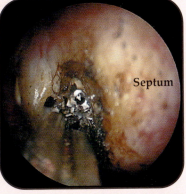

The sphenoidotomy is enlarged sufficiently for intrasphenoid evaluation and disease removal. This opening must be connected to the natural ostium.

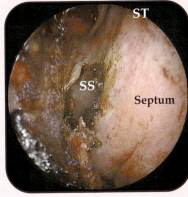 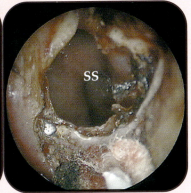

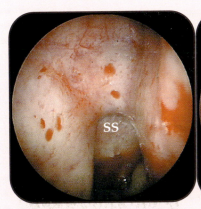 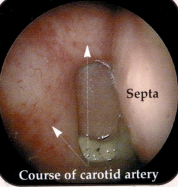 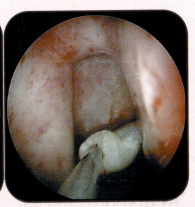

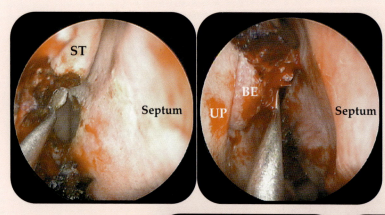

An angled curette is used to open the posterior ethmoid cell, which is in front of the anterior wall of the sphenoid.

After the recesses of the posterior ethmoid cells are felt, the septa are resected with the angled curette by making movements in the anteroinferior direction.

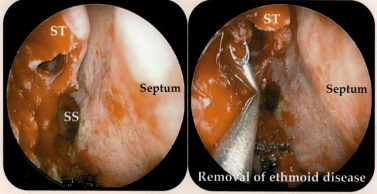

The roof of the posterior ethmoid is identified and the mucosa over the roof is preserved. The curette dissection is continued until the posterior ethmoid cavity is sufficiently exteriorized.

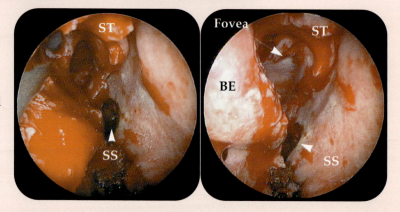

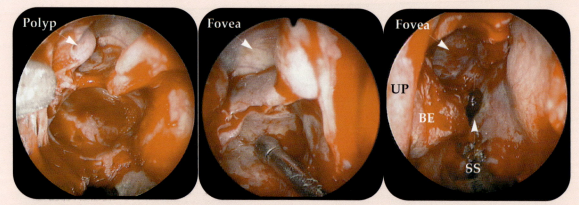

Dissection is limited to the posterior ethmoid. The procedure is terminated by placing rolled gel film and applying Bactroban ointment.

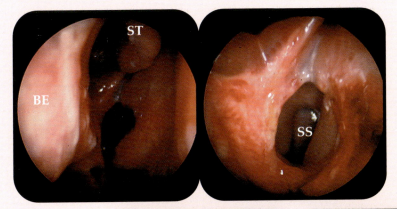

This four-week postoperative view shows beautiful healing. The sphenoid and ethmoid cavities are patent. The intact bulla and uncinate indicate the integrity of the anterior ethmoid as a result of the minimally invasive technique. Six months postoperatively the patient is asymptomatic and disease free.

Six-month postoperative view. Observe the shrinkage of the sphenoid ostium.

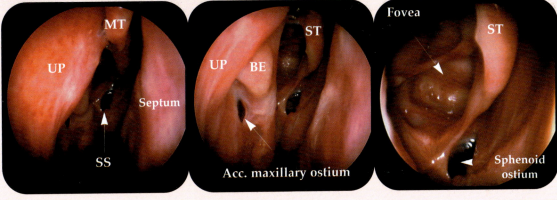

Pansinusitis with Polyposis (Group III B)
Recurring sinusitis with CT evidence of disease in one or two sinuses
(sphenoethmoid disease with frontal sinuses opacity)

This 38-year-old woman presented with a three-year history of sinus disease symptoms with intermittent treatment. Extensive bilateral pansinusitis with involvement of the sphenoethmoid recesses and sphenoid sinuses is evident on the CT scan below. Endoscopic evaluation revealed bilateral polyposis (these polyps were nonallergenic as no specific allergen was detected by RAST and skin testing). A transethmoid sphenoidotomy was performed. Resection of the disease from the anterior to the posterior direction in such cases affords better visualization of the sphenoethmoid recess. The polyps were resected with the KTP laser, exposing the uncinate plate. The subsequent surgical steps are as described on pages 123 through 125.

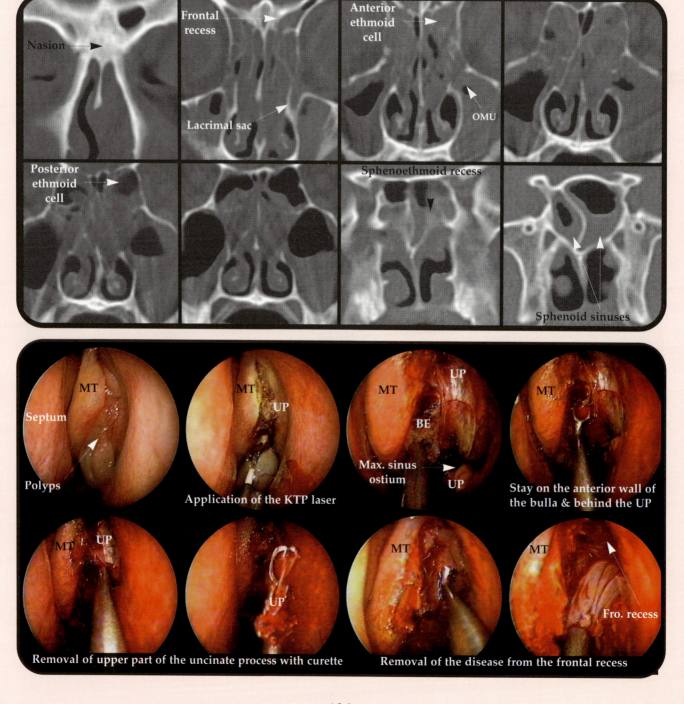

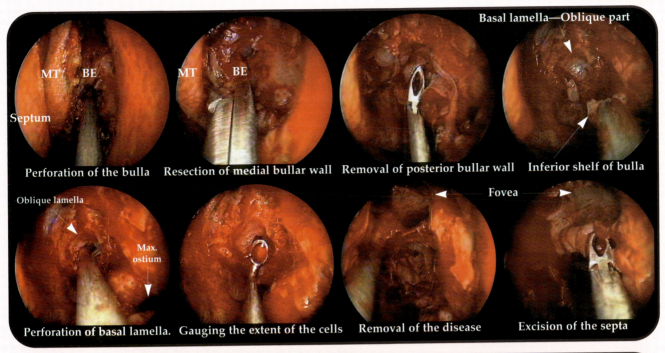

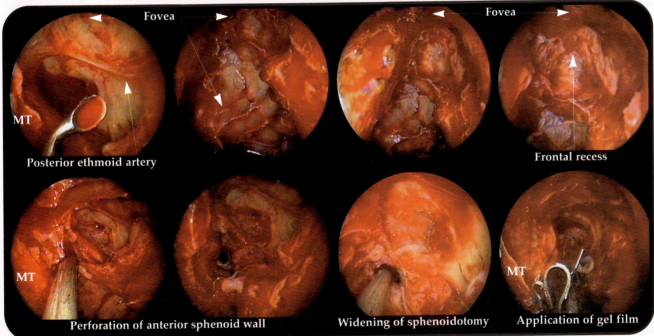

Three-month postoperative endoscopic views

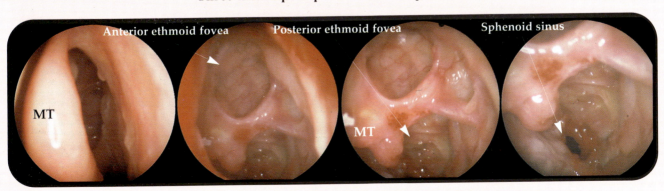

Revision Sphenoidotomy (Group III A)

Recurring sinusitis with CT evidence of disease in one or two sinuses (sphenoethmoid disease with clear frontal sinuses)

Common causes of postoperative recurrence of sphenoid disease are:
- Failure to connect the sphenoidotomy to the natural ostium during surgery.
- Persistence or recurrence of posterior ethmoid disease.
- Postoperative adhesions causing blockage of the sphenoethmoid recess.

The management of such a recurrence depends on the underlying cause. CT evaluation of the lamina papyracea, the fovea, the optic nerve and the internal carotid artery is of paramount importance before any surgical intervention. The aim in performing revision surgery is to reestablish the drainage system by widening the sphenoethmoid recess, connecting the sphenoidotomy to the natural ostium and removing disease from the posterior ethmoid, if present. The sphenoethmoid recess can be widened laterally by resecting the superior turbinate, posterior part of the middle turbinate and posterior ethmoid as necessary. However, when the posterior ethmoid is disease free, I prefer not to violate it. It is preferable to resect the sphenoid rostrum medially to obtain the desired effect. In my opinion, the KTP/532 laser is the ideal instrument for this procedure.

The following case illustrates a revision sphenoidotomy in an 11-year-old patient. An endoscopic sphenoidotomy with marsupialization of a large mucocele and a nasal septum reconstruction were the primary procedures. A very narrow sphenoethmoid recess and inability to debride in the office setting resulted in a recurrence. The surgical steps are depicted below.

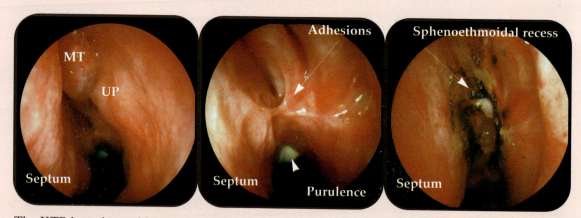

The KTP laser is used in the near-contact mode at 10 to 12 watts of power to vaporize the adhesions.

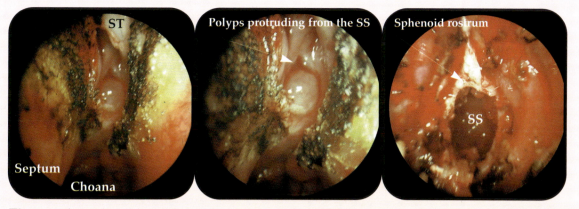

The anterior sphenoid wall is lased, the sphenoidotomy is completed, and the scars between the sphenoid and superior turbinate are resected. The polypoid disease is debrided. Medially the rostrum is resected. This creates a 1-cm opening in the posterosuperior part of the septum.

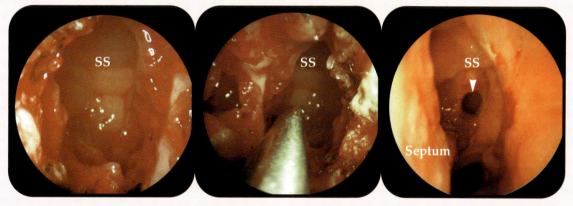

The above photographs show inflamed sphenoid mucosa, resected sphenoid rostrum and healing sphenoidotomy.

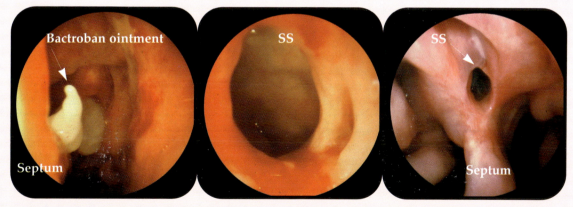

Postoperatively, debridement and application of Bactroban ointment is continued until healing is complete. Five years postoperatively the patient remains symptom free and no whistling resulted from the resection of the rostrum.

9
Minimally Invasive Techniques in Pediatric Sinus Diseases

The principles of minimally invasive techniques as discussed in the previous chapters hold just as true for children.
- Minimal surgical trauma.
- Preservation of natural anatomy.
- Reestablishment of ventilation.

The above basic tenets should be very strictly adhered to when dealing with the pediatric population. The following table of sinusitis should be helpful in investigating the cases and planning the surgery. If surgery is inevitable, it should be performed by a surgeon who is familiar with pediatric anatomy.

Sinusitis

Purulent	Nonpurulent	Secondary to genetic disorders
Sinusitis as a result of: • Frequent upper respiratory infections • Recurring adenotonsillitis • Foreign bodies	Obstructive sinusitis as a result of: • Mucocele • Polyps	• Cystic fibrosis • Primary ciliary dyskinesia (PCD)

Investigations
- Culture and sensitivity of nasal and/or pharyngeal discharges
- Allergy investigations, especially in cases of negative throat cultures
- Work-up for immunodeficiency: total immunoglobulins and IgG subclasses
- CT scan of paranasal sinuses
- Sinus x-rays and lateral view of the nasopharynx for adenoidal hypertrophy
- Work-up for genetic disorders: sweat chloride, DNA study and nasal mucosal biopsy for ciliary study

Conservative treatment
- Culture-based prolonged antibiotic courses (21-day course repeated at 2-week interval)
- Avoid exposure
- Allergy treatment
- Consider pneumoccal vaccine

Surgical management

• Adenoidectomy • Tonsilloadenoidectomy • Removal of foreign body	• Conchoplasty or middle turbinoplasty • Septoplasty	• OMU reconstruction • Caldwell-Luc with resection of polyps without injury to OMU	• Total ethmoidectomy • OMU reconstruction

The importance of the anatomical configuration of all sinuses in children lies partly in their size. Because they are much smaller, there is less room for manipulation and a greater chance of complications. The use of small-sized pediatric instruments, 2.7-mm endoscope, microdebrider and KTP/532 laser is of special advantage here. Gentle manipulation and the least possible surgical trauma should be the main aim. It is critical to evaluate the ethmoid infundibulum and identify the diseased maxillary ostium. The KTP laser with its small tip (0.6 mm) and the flexibility of its fiber permits access into very narrow niches. Its hemostatic capabilities provide a relatively dry surgical field. In addition, the laser enables a partial uncinectomy with preservation of the inner mucosal lining of the infundibulum better than any other instrument. This reduces the incidence of maxillary ostial stenosis and injury to the lamina papyracea and the frontal recess.

On the other hand the new generation microdebrider with its suction port also allows good visulization. However, in order to use the microdebrider, one must perform a partial uncinectomy first. Refer to pages 95 through 97.

Before any surgical intervention, it is vital to study the CT anatomy of the sinuses. The details of development and anatomy are discussed in Chapter 3. The following CT scan depicts the normal configuration of the sinuses at the age of 1 year. The salient features seen are:
- Absence of frontal sinuses.
- Prominent and well-developed agger cells.
- Well-formed maxillary sinuses. Note that the maxillary floor is at a higher level than the nasal floor.
- Small posterior ethmoid cells.
- Just developing sphenoid sinuses.

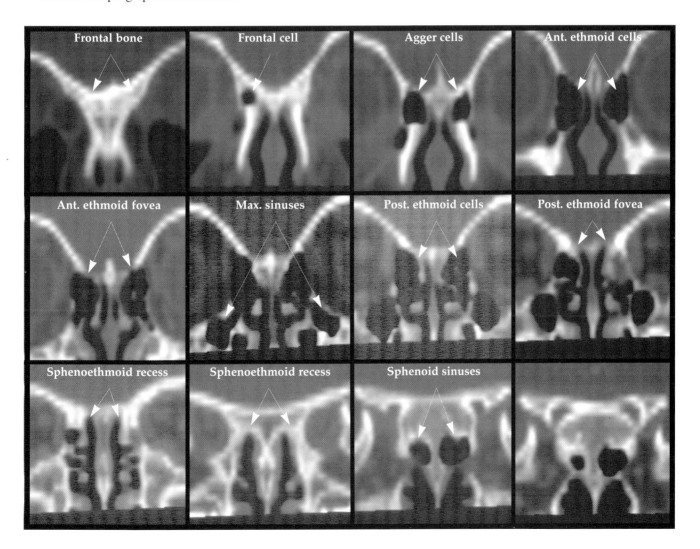

The following case depicts the management of nonpurulent obstructive sinusitis resulting from a large antrochoanal polyp in an 8-year-old child. The pharyngeal cultures were negative on two occasions. Endonasal examination revealed a large polyp obstructing the nose. The CT scan shows pneumatized frontal sinuses, clear agger cell and frontal recess, complete opacification of the right maxillary sinus with widening of the infundibulum and partial opacification of the anterior and posterior ethmoid and sphenoid sinuses.

Sinusitis cases of this type should be handled with extreme care. Removal of the obstructing polyp from the ostiomeatal unit usually results in resolution of disease in all sinuses. It is better to take a conservative approach, as shown.

Preoperative CT scan

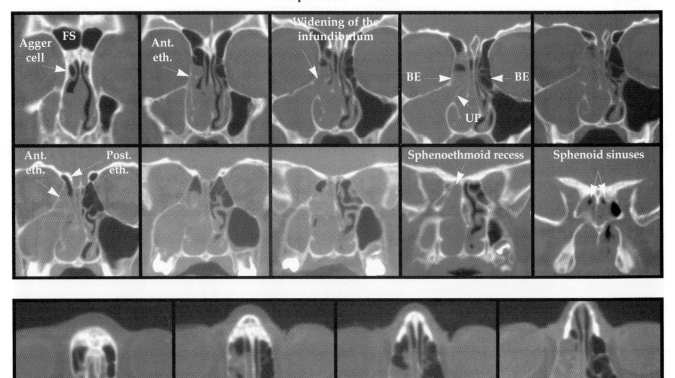

Six-month postoperative CT scan

Generally, a postoperative CT scan is not necessary if the patient is asymptomatic. In children, however, it is advisable because postoperative endonasal evaluation is difficult and inaccurate. In this case the child was completely asymptomatic. The CT scan, however, reveals a small mucosal polyp in the maxillary floor. The remaining sinuses show complete resolution of disease. Since the patient is asymptomatic, no further surgical intervention is planned.

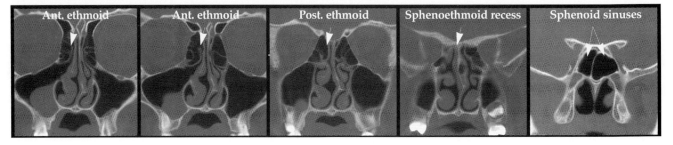

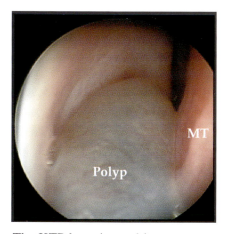 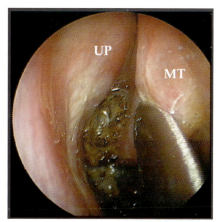 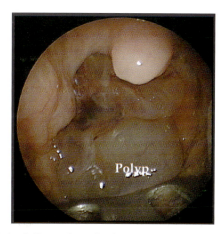

The KTP laser is used in a near-contact technique to resect the polyp, which is delivered orally because of its large size.

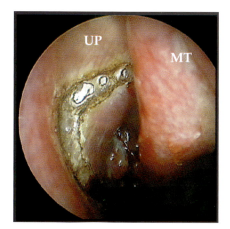 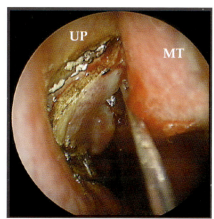 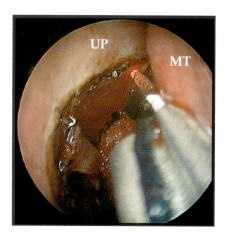

The uncinate process is defined and its inferior half is resected, keeping the inner infundibular mucosal lining intact. Nick's triangle technique is used for accurate identification of the maxillary ostium. An inner mucosal flap is created and reflected inferiorly over the inferior turbinate.

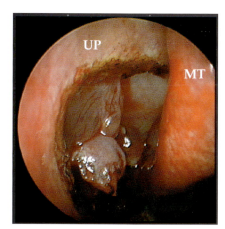 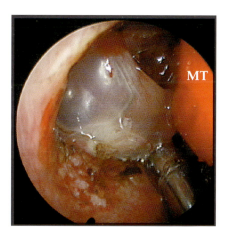 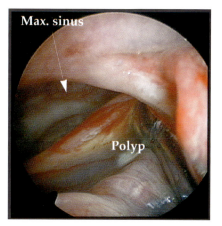

The maxillary ostium has been widened by the expanding polyp, which is resected with a giraffe forceps, preserving a maximum amount of the mucosal lining.

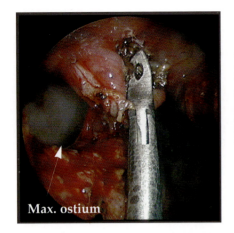

Max. ostium

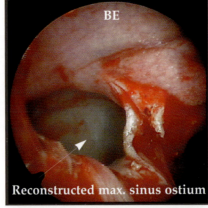

BE

Reconstructed max. sinus ostium

Excess mucosa from the flap is trimmed with the Thru-Cut forceps.

A window was created in the bulla ethmoidalis that revealed clear mucus and hypertrophic mucosa. No further resection was performed. The surgery is completed with application of Bactroban ointment. The nose was not packed.

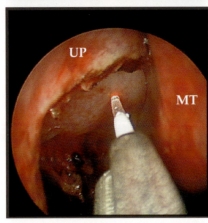

UP, MT

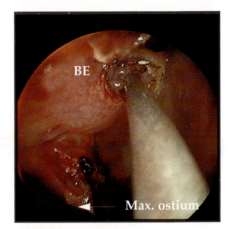

BE, Max. ostium

The following case illustrates chronic purulent sinusitis and its management in a 9-year-old child. The patient had undergone tonsilloadenoidectomy and bilateral tympanostomy tube placement for chronic bilateral serous otitis media. After extrusion of the tubes, the symptoms recurred. On further investigations, bilateral pansinusitis was detected on the CT scan, as shown below. A complete allergy work-up was negative. After three months of intense culture-driven antibiotic courses, a repeat CT scan revealed an increase in the disease process, as shown below.

First preoperative CT scan

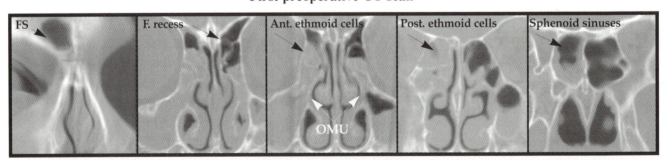

Second preoperative CT scan

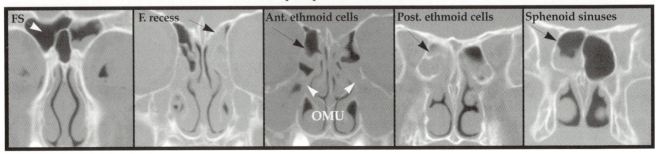

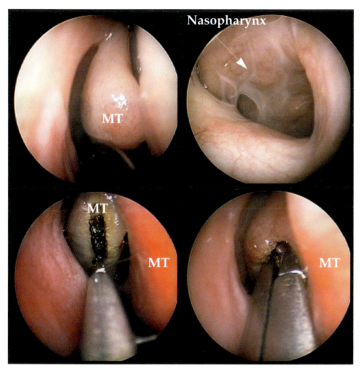

On endoscopy, purulent discharge was seen in the middle meatus and in the nasopharynx. The middle turbinate was bony, so I elected to perform submucous turbinoplasty with maximum mucosal preservation. An incision was made on the inferior surface of the turbinate mucosa and a subperiosteal flap created. A part of the turbinate bone was resected and the subperiosteal flap draped back.

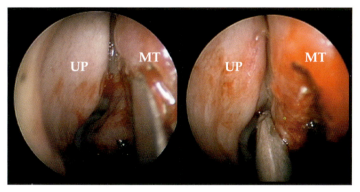

Next, the uncinate process was anchored by the probe and its mobile part defined by wiggling it. This is an important step for planning the incision for uncinectomy.

The inferior half of the uncinate process was resected using the Nick's triangle technique. The KTP laser was used to resect the uncinate process layer by layer, resulting in maximal mucosal preservation of the infundibulum. A relatively dry field was maintained, which facilitated identification of the diseased maxillary ostium. As opposed to this, the pediatric back-biter will resect a considerable amount of the infundibular mucosa and cause bleeding, putting the surgeon at a disadvantage.

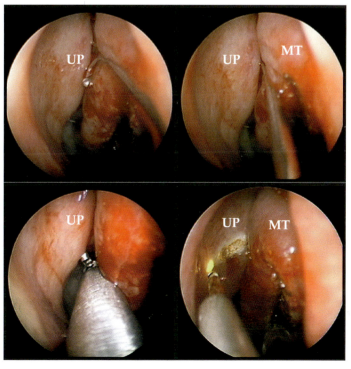

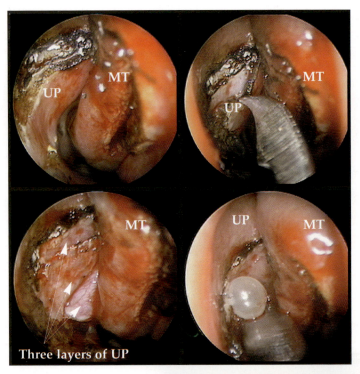

These surgical photographs demonstrate the technique of partial uncinectomy:
- Incision on the mucosa of the uncinate process.
- Elevation of the mucosa and separation of the bony uncinate plate.
- Creation of the inner infundibular mucosal flap.
- A bubble with mucopus is seen emerging from the maxillary ostium.

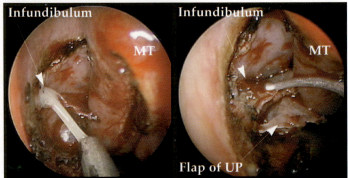

- Removal of mucopus.
- Identification of the maxillary ostium with a ball probe sliding over the inner mucosal lining.
- Widening of the maxillary ostium by submucosal removal of the remaining bony uncinate plate.
- Draping of the inner mucosal flap over the inferior turbinate.

Note:
The uncinate process has three layers: the inner mucosal layer, the middle bony layer and the outer mucosal layer. The inner mucosal layer is also the medial mucosal wall of the infundibulum.

In performing a partial uncinectomy the inner mucosal layer is very carefully preserved and reflected inferiorly over the inferior turbinate.

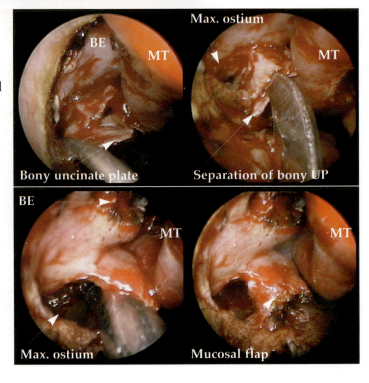

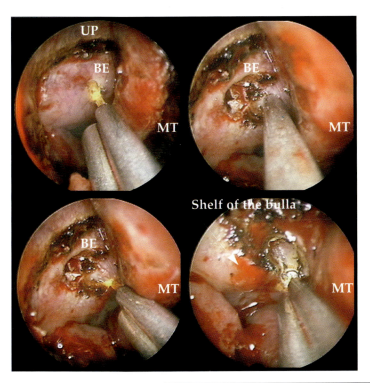

- Creation of a window in the bulla with the KTP laser.
- Clear bulla ethmoidalis.
- Creation of a window in the posterior ethmoid through the oblique part of the basal lamella.
- Clear posterior ethmoid cell.

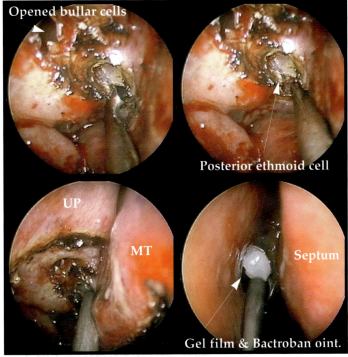

The above case is an ideal example of the application of minimally invasive technique. Although the CT scan revealed marked disease in most sinuses, at surgery the disease was limited to the ostiomeatal unit. Windows created in the bulla and the posterior ethmoid did not reveal significant disease in those areas. Hence total ethmoid resection was avoided. In such cases, if the disease recurs, a second stage procedure can be performed.

10

ADJUVANT PROCEDURES

Endoscopic Pituitary Surgery

Indications
I. Pituitary adenomas
   A. Functioning
      1. Excessive secretion of growth hormone—acromegaly
      2. Excess secretion of ACTH hormone—Cushing's syndrome (chromophobe or basophilic)
      3. Hyposecretory—uncommon
   B. Nonfunctioning

II. Nonpituitary disorders
   A. Metastatic tumors
   B. Neural tumors—glioma, meningioma
   C. Cell rest tumors—chordoma, craniopharyngioma, cholesteatoma, keratoma
   D. Sphenoid sinus disorders—mucocele, granuloma
   E. Empty sella

Contraindications
Aneurysm of internal carotid artery; conchal-type sphenoid sinus (relative contraindiction).

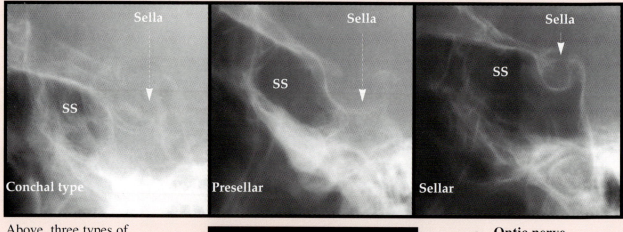

Above, three types of pneumatization

Surgical Anatomy

Refer to pages 48 through 51.

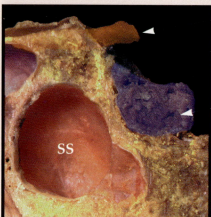

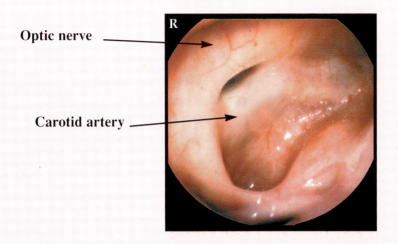

MRI Anatomy and Tumor

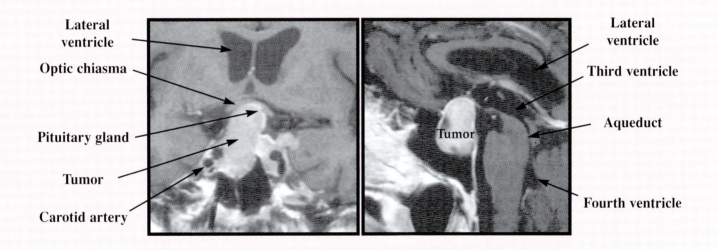

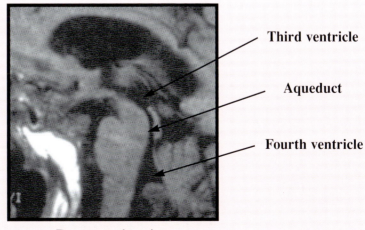

Postoperative view

Technique of Endoscopic Transseptal Transsphenoidal Hypophysectomy

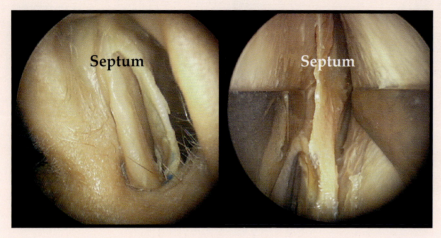

- Make a complete or hemitransfixation incision.
- Elevate a mucoperichondrial flap of the cartilaginous septum on one side.
- Elevate mucoperiosteal flaps on both sides of the bony septum up to the sphenoid rostrum.
- Separate the cartilaginous septum inferiorly from the maxillary crest and posteriorly from the vomer and the perpendicular plate of the ethmoid.

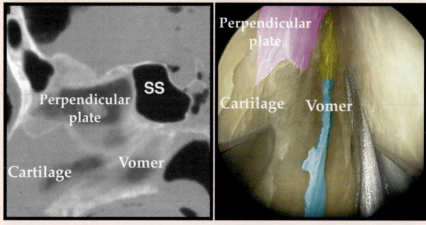

- Remove the posterosuperior part of the perpendicular plate of the ethmoid and the upper half of the vomer to expose the sphenoid rostrum.

- Elevate the mucoperiosteal flaps of the anterior wall of the sphenoid.
- Identify the sphenoid ostium on each side.
- Make a sphenoidotomy on either side at the ostium or just below the ostium, close to the midline.
- Resect part of the rostrum.

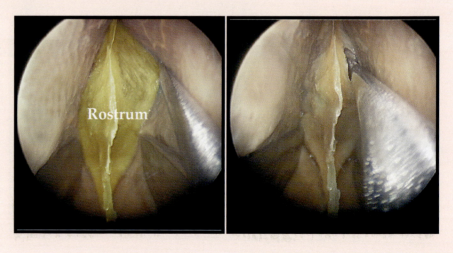

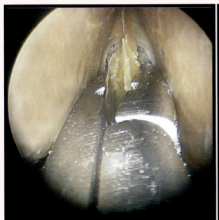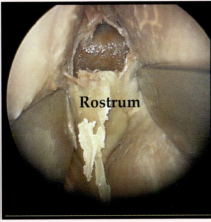

- Enlarge the sphenoidotomy laterally as far as the lateral bony wall, using the sphenoid punch under direct vision.
- Remove the overhang of the anterior bony wall, with careful identification of the sphenoid roof.
- Evaluate the intrasphenoidal space and the anatomical landmarks with a ball probe.
- Before resecting the sphenoid septa, observe their position on an axial CT scan.

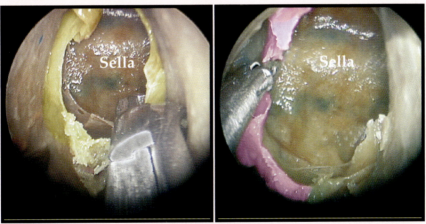

- Confirm the attachment of the sphenoid septa. Be careful: check to see if any septa are connected to the carotid artery or the optic nerve.
- Resect in very small bites with the Thru-Cut forceps.

- Identify the sella turcica.
- Elevate the mucosa of the sella.
- Fracture the sella in an eggshell fashion and remove bony fragments with a 2-mm pituitary forceps.

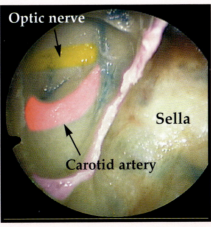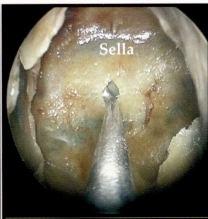

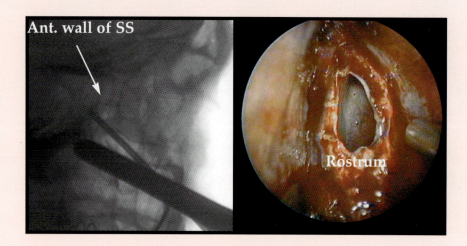

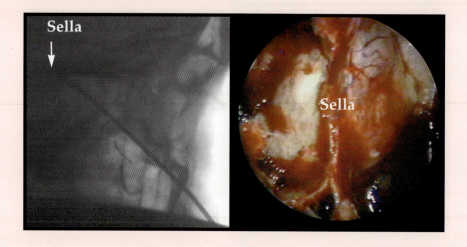

- Electrocauterize the dura over the pituitary tumor (bipolar or suction cautery).
- Incise the dura.
- Biopsy the tumor with pituitary forceps—confirm with a frozen section.
- Debulk the tumor with a blunt ring curette.

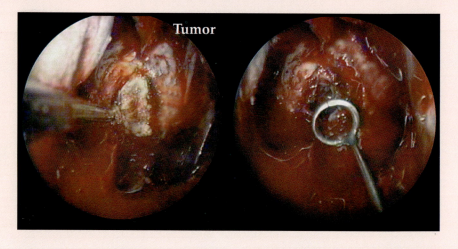

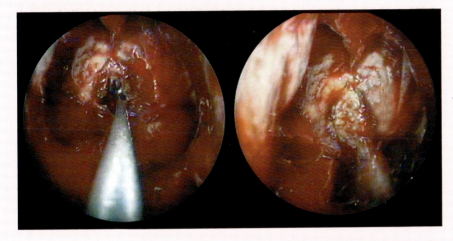

- Remove the residual tumor with a blunt ring curette. Try to keep the capsule intact.

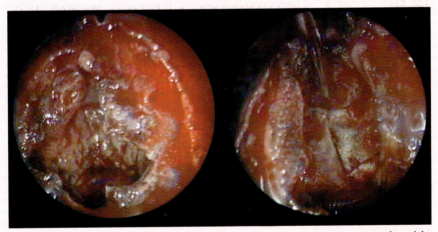

- Evaluate the lateral and superior recesses inside the tumor capsule with a 30-degree endoscope.

- Fill the capsule with fat or fascia.
- Apply fibrin glue.
- Apply a piece of cartilage or bone (from the septum) to support the tissue seal.
- Reconstruct the septum.
- Apply septal splints on either side.

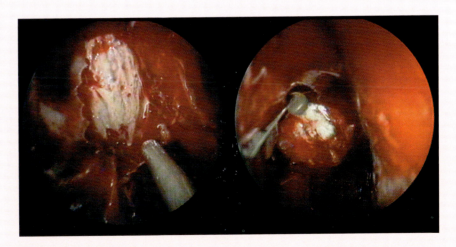

Endoscopic Dacryocystorhinostomy—Primary and Revision

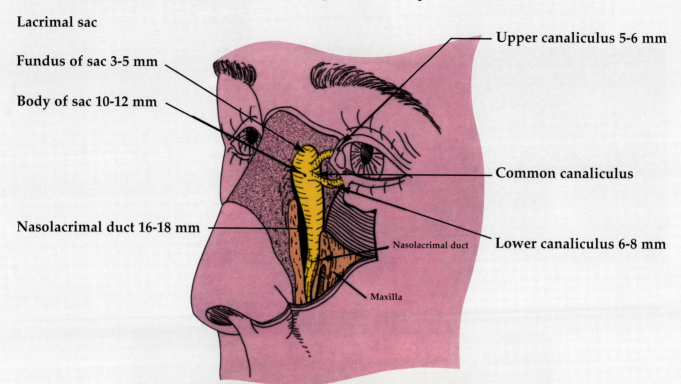

- Lacrimal sac
- Fundus of sac 3-5 mm
- Body of sac 10-12 mm
- Nasolacrimal duct 16-18 mm
- Upper canaliculus 5-6 mm
- Common canaliculus
- Lower canaliculus 6-8 mm
- Nasolacrimal duct
- Maxilla

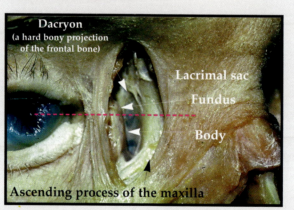

Dacryon (a hard bony projection of the frontal bone); Lacrimal sac Fundus, Body; Ascending process of the maxilla

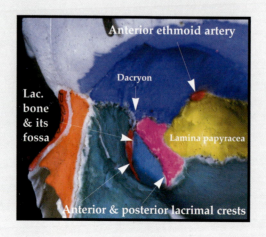

Anterior ethmoid artery; Dacryon; Lac. bone & its fossa; Lamina papyracea; Anterior & posterior lacrimal crests

- In this cadaveric dissection, the medial canthal tendon has been removed, revealing the superior and nasal extent of the lacrimal sac.
- The key to a successful endoscopic DCR is identification of the full extent of the lacrimal sac. Since the ascending process of the maxilla shields part of the sac, it becomes necessary to shave off part of the ascending process until the entire anterior extent of the sac can be identified.
- Next, the lacrimal bone is resected to expose the entire sac intranasally.
- The above bone resections ensure a large fenestrum. The larger the opening, the better the outcome. The average size should be 1 x 1.5 cm.
- After full intranasal exposure of the sac, its entire medial wall is resected.

- The canaliculi and the sac are intubated with silicon tubing. The tube is removed when the intranasal healing is complete, in 4 to 8 weeks.
- The KTP/532 laser is used:
  1. To strip the mucosa over the ascending process of the maxilla.
  2. To resect the part of uncinate process over the lacrimal sac and the lacrimal bone.
  3. To obtain hemostasis. The relatively dry field enables precise identification of the landmarks.
- The laser should not be used to resect the sac, nor should it be passed through the canaliculus because the scatter effect (produced by all lasers) is most undesirable in such small structures. It can result in scarring and adhesions.

Indications
Obstruction of the lacrimal sac, common canaliculus or nasolacrimal duct. Recurring dacryocystitis or stones in the sac.

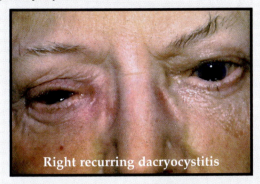
Right recurring dacryocystitis

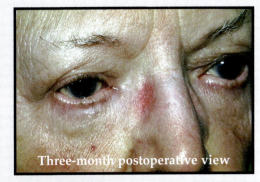
Three-month postoperative view

History Taking

A. Eye and general
1. Tearing: Unilateral or bilateral?
2. Tearing: Constant or episodic?
3. History of dacryocystitis?
4. History of trauma or surgery?
5. History of allergy or irritation?
6. Any underlying eye disease?
7. Any related systematic disease, e.g., thyroid disorder, arthritis?
8. Congenital malformation?

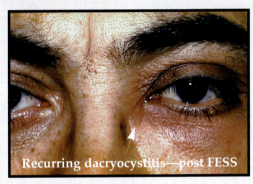
Recurring dacryocystitis—post FESS

B. Nasal
1. Any nasal obstruction? Unilateral or bilateral?
2. Rhinorrhea? Sinus pressure or pain?
3. History of nasal sinus surgery? Is tearing on the same side as above symptoms?

Concepts

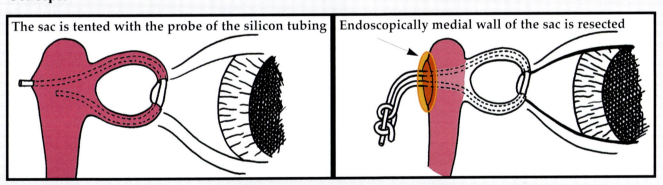

The sac is tented with the probe of the silicon tubing | Endoscopically medial wall of the sac is resected

The concept of this surgery is to connect the lacrimal sac directly with the nasal cavity with minimal trauma.

The general area in which the lacrimal bone is removed during the intranasal dacryocystorhinostomy is outlined.

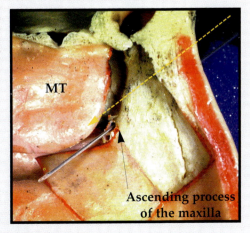
MT
Ascending process of the maxilla

On the lateral wall of the nose at the level of the anterior border of the middle turbinate, a bony ridge is seen and felt. This ridge is the internal representation of the ascending process of the maxilla. Posterior to this is the lacrimal groove. In order to visualize the lacrimal sac fully, it is imperative to thin out this ascending process after resecting the mucosa. It is best done with the power drill.

Instruments and Materials

- Lacrimal dilators.
- Lacrimal probes.
- Lacrimal cannula, 23 G.
- Schirmer test strips.
- Fluorescein dye.
- Ophthaine, local anesthetic eyedrops.
- Saline eyewash.

Instruments and Materials

The following are my preferences:
- Lacrimal dilator made by Storz, Cat. # E 4340
- Lacrimal cannula, 23 G Storz, Cat. # E 4410

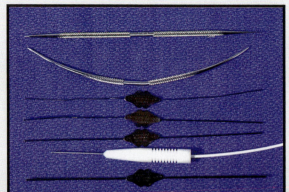

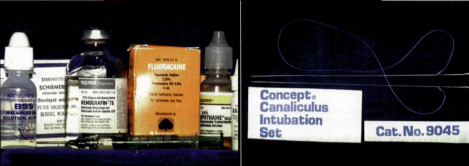

Light Pipe.
Order from:
Grieshaber & Co.
3000 Cabot Boulevard West
Langhome, PA 19047
Tel. (215) 741-0550

Concept Canaliculus Intubation Set.
Order from:
CONCEPT Inc.,
11311 Concept Blvd.
Largo, FL 34643.

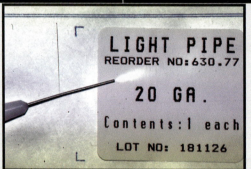

Diagnostic Tests and Radiological Identification of the Lacrimal Sac

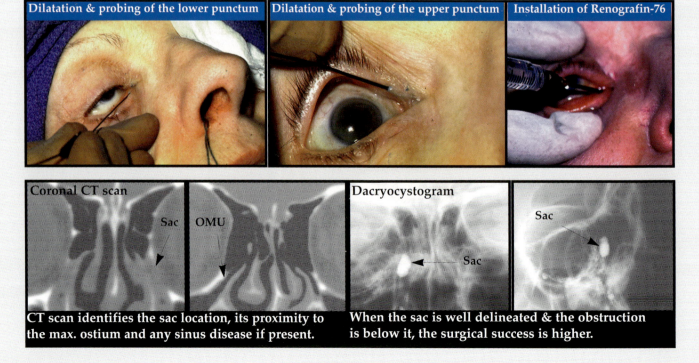

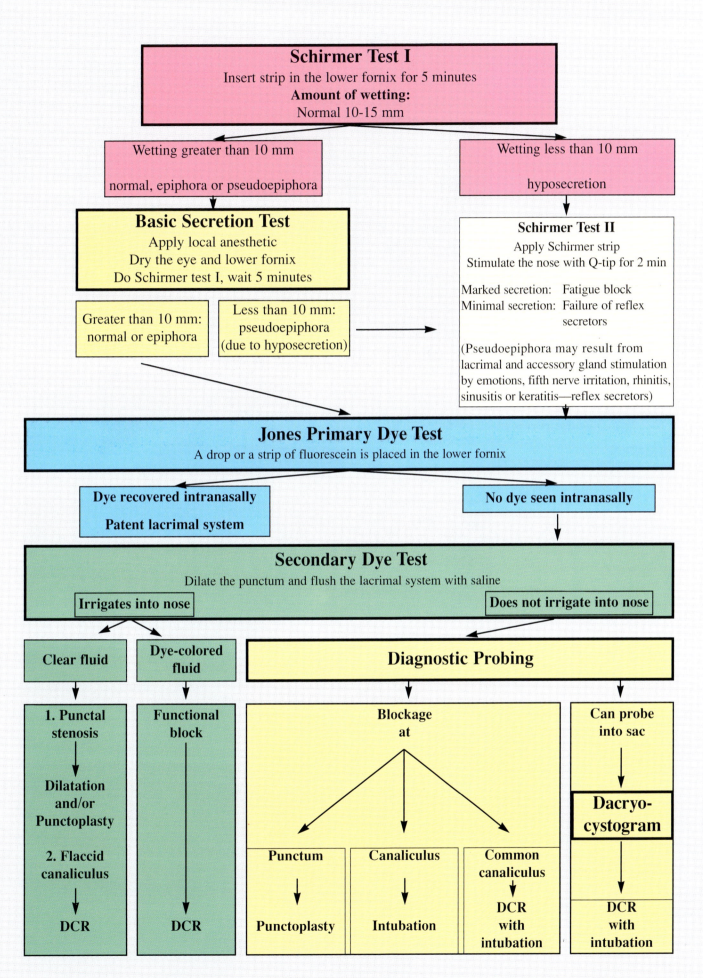

Surgical Technique

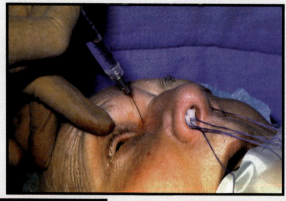

Anesthesia
- Local or general.
- Nasal application of cottonoids soaked with 2% Pontocaine and Oxymetazoline.
- Lacrimal block by injection with 1% Xylocaine with epinephrine (1:100,000).
- Intranasal block with the same solution.

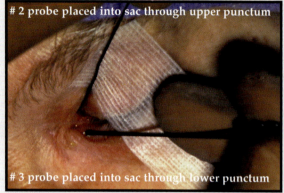

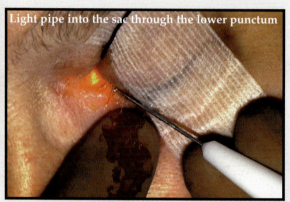

Both puncta are dilated. Pass the # 3 probe into the sac through the inferior punctum. If the light pipe is available it is lubricated and inserted into the sac. It is imperative that the direction of the light probe be medial and inferior, pointing toward the nasal spine. Stabilize the light probe in this position and protect the eye with a wet gauze sponge. In order to see the transilluminated area well, reduce the endoscopic light.

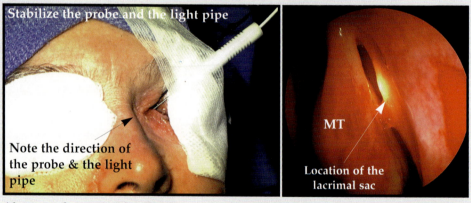

Absence of agger nasi cell allows good transillumination delineating the sac.

In this case a large agger nasi cell obstructs the transilluminated light from the light probe. Studies indicate that in approximately 40% of patients the ethmoid air cells extend into the ascending process of the maxilla. In approximately 53% of cases, agger nasi cells will extend anteriorly to the posterior lacrimal crest. Hence, in over 90% cases, the surgeon will encounter the ethmoid air cells prior to reaching the lacrimal sac.

The mucosa over the ascending process is stripped off. Here the KTP laser is used.

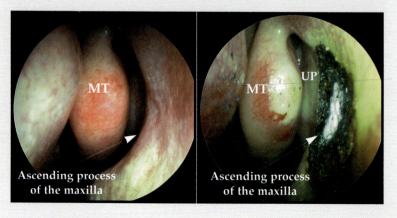

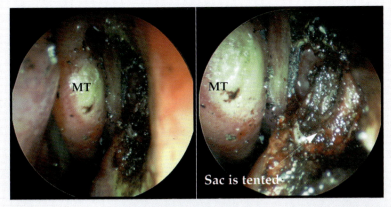

The sickle knife is used to open the lacrimal sac. Its entire medial wall is excised with the Thru-Cut forceps so that a fistula of adequate size is formed. The excised part of the lacrimal sac is submitted for histopathological examination.

The canaliculi and the sac are intubated and the tubes are tied in the nasal cavity. Antibacterial ointment is applied at the site.

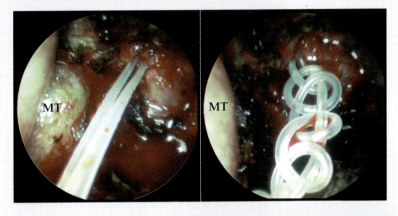

Postoperative care
1. Refrain from blowing the nose till the healing is complete.
2. Saline nasal spray.
3. Periodic endoscopic debridement.
4. Remove the silicone tube when the healing is complete (six to eight weeks).

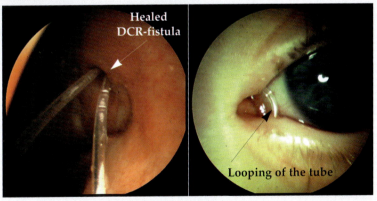

In some cases during the surgical procedure the lacrimal fossa may be difficult to identify. If this happens, in order to verify the lacrimal fossa, first palpate it externally. Then place the J-curette externally along the side of the nose on the fossa and measure the distance to the nasal spine as shown here. Then move the curette intranasally and use the measurement to locate the area of the fossa. One must be able to palpate the curette bimanually. This will verify the adequacy of lacrimal bone resection.

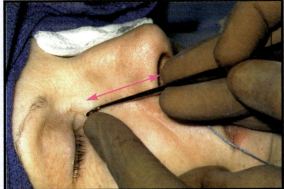
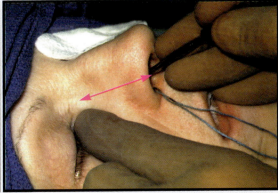

Revision Dacryocystorhinostomy—Office Procedure

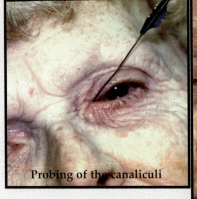

Probing of the canaliculi

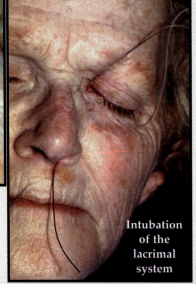

Intubation of the lacrimal system

If, as mentioned before, the lacrimal sac fenestration is large enough, the success rate of this procedure is very high—above 90%. In case of recurrence, however, a revision procedure can be done under local anesthesia in the office or as outpatient surgery.

Under local anesthesia, both canaliculi are probed to break up the scar tissue and adhesions. Intubation is performed and left in place for six months. After removal of the tubes, local massage is continued in an effort to keep the passage open.

If adequate bone removal is not done the first time, the patient may have to be reoperated on under local or general anesthesia for the proper amount of bone resection, as shown on the opposite page.

Any other obstruction, e.g., turbinate, if present, should also be resected. In all cases of revision surgery, the silicon tubing should be kept in place for a longer period of time.

If all revision procedures fail, the last resort is a conjunctivodacryocystorhinostomy (bypassing the sac) performed with the ophthalmologist.

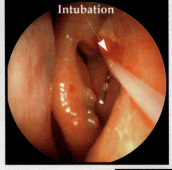

Reestablishing DCR-fistula

Intubation

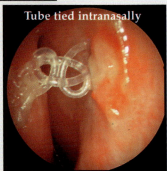

Tube tied intranasally

Complications of DCR
1. Granuloma. Treat with local debridement and application of antibacterial ointment.
2. Stenosis. Treat with reintubation.
3. Injury to the eye.
4. Allergic reaction to the silicon tubing. Treat with removal of the tube.
5. Periorbital surgical emphysema. Treat with application of ice, watchful waiting and having patient refrain from blowing the nose until the healing is complete.

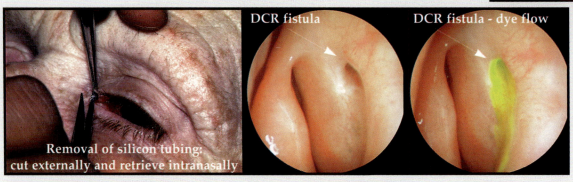

Removal of silicon tubing: cut externally and retrieve intranasally

DCR fistula

DCR fistula - dye flow

Six-month postoperative views showing a patent DCR fistula after removal of the silicone tubing.

Revision Dacryocystorhinostomy—Formal Procedure

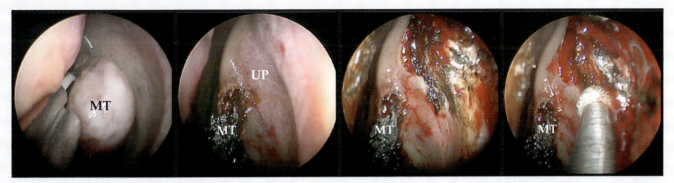

Partial turbinotomy exposing the operative area.

Removal of mucosa and thinning of the ascending process.

Further resection of the ascending process of maxilla.

Superior extent of dissection. KTP laser resection of the thin lacrimal bone.

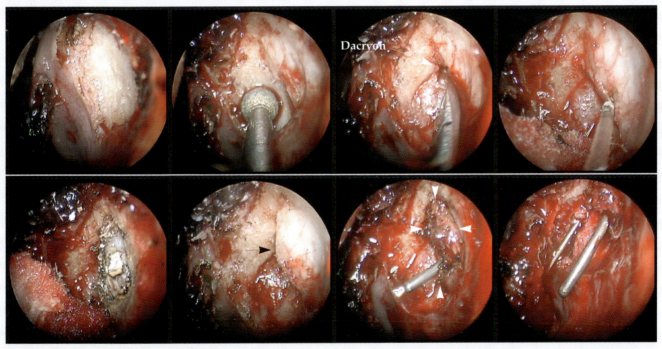

Removal of the lacrimal bone and tenting the lacrimal sac.

Extent of resection of the medial wall of the lacrimal sac.

Intubation of the lacrimal system.

Left, antibiotic application; right, postoperative view showing the flow of the fluorescein dye from the DCR fistula.

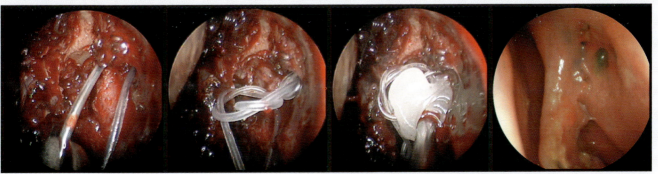

Orbital Decompression

Indications

Graves' ophthalmopathy.

Orbital decompression is performed in cases of Graves' ophthalmopathy with malignant exophthalmos. This is associated with a thyroid disorder, but there is no proportionate relationship between the two. Orbital decompression is indicated when the progression of the exophthalmos is rapid and vision is threatened. The purpose is to provide more space for the swollen tissues to relieve the orbital tissue tension. This decompresses the optic nerve, thus restoring vision, and allows extraocular muscles to function and the lids to close. Cosmetically, it improves the appearance.

Pathology

Proptosis results from an increase in the amount of orbital fat and interstitial edema of extraocular muscles. If unchecked, the muscles undergo degenerative changes that result in restriction of ocular movement. Boggy and swollen tissues compress the optic nerve, resulting in visual loss. Corneal exposure due to inability to close the lids results in keratopathy. Infections may lead to further damage and loss of vision.

Surgical Technique

Ideally, this procedure is performed with an ophthalmologist. It is done under local or general anesthesia. Meticulous hemostasis should be maintained throughout the surgery. Avoid injury to the frontal recess and the lacrimal system anteriorly and to the optic nerve posteriorly. The maxillary sinus ostium is enlarged sufficiently to accommodate the protruding orbital contents and to prevent obstructive maxillary sinusitis. The orbital fat should be handled gently during the procedure and care should be taken to avoid injury to the rectus muscles. At the conclusion of the procedure, adequacy of the decompression should be evaluated by palpating the orbit while observing endoscopically. Following are the surgical steps.

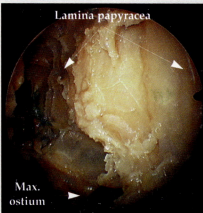

Complete sphenoethmoidectomy with delineation of the entire bony plate of the lamina papyracea.

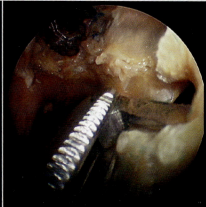

Enlargement of the maxillary ostium at the expense of the anteroinferior fontanelle, with care taken not to injure the nasolacrimal duct.

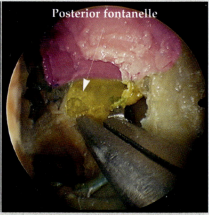

Enlargement of the maxillary ostium at the expense of the posterior fontanelle all the way to the posterior wall of the maxillary sinus.

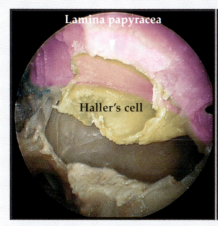
Identification and removal of Haller's cell if present.

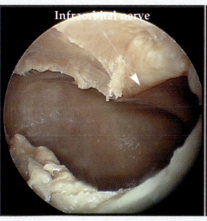
Dissection and exposure of the roof of the maxillary sinus until the infraorbital nerve is identified.

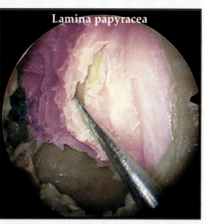
Separation and removal of the bony lamina papyracea from the orbital periosteum. A small anterosuperior segment is preserved at the agger nasi to maintain the integrity of the frontal recess.

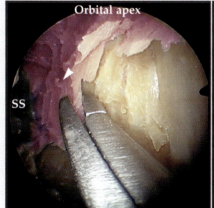
Continued separation and removal of the lamina papyracea posteriorly toward the orbital apex.

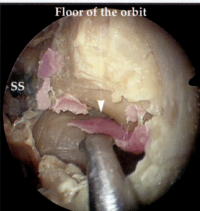
Resection of the bony orbital floor medial to the infraorbital nerve.

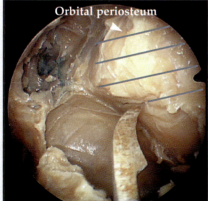
Incisions made on the orbital periosteum directed posteroanteriorly, starting at the lateral side and continuing medially and upward. This prevents obscuration of the surgical field by dripping blood and the herniating orbital fat.

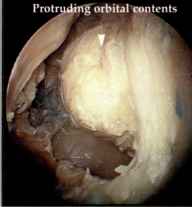
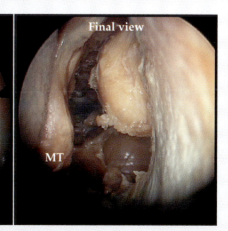
Shown is maximum herniation of the orbital contents into the maxillary sinus and the middle meatus.

Osteoma

A middle-aged woman was seen with complaints of left orbital and facial pain and nasal congestion of six months' duration. She was referred by a neurologist based on an MRI scan that showed left maxillary sinusitis. CT revealed an osteoma of the ethmoid that was attached to the lamina cribrosa. There was thickening of the mucoperiosteum of the maxillary sinus and bullar cell, and the nasal septum was deviated to the left with a lateralized middle turbinate. Endoscopic evaluation in the office was not fruitful, as the middle meatus could not be visualized.

Surgical Technique

When the operative space is compromised by the deviated nasal septum, it is imperative to reconstruct the septum before starting the sinus surgical procedure. This is done to clearly define the frontal recess and fovea and to minimize tissue injury.

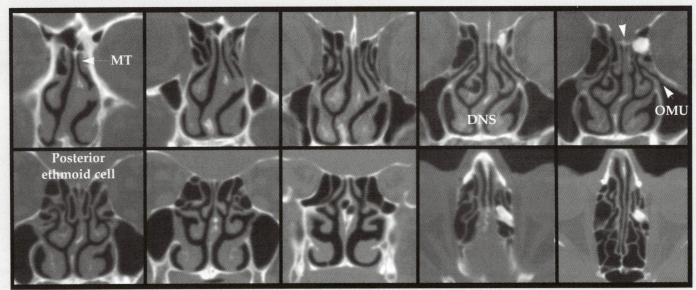

The endoscopic view here shows a thin, delicate middle turbinate that is lateralized, compressing the middle meatus. In order to approach the ethmoid, most surgeons medialize the middle turbinate. This invariably results in fracture of the vertical lamella, an unstable middle turbinate, further lateralization, and postoperatively an obstructed middle meatus. Manipulation of the vertical lamella should be avoided altogether. I use the KTP/532 laser with 600-micron fibers in a near-contact technique with continuous lasing at 12 watts of power to resect the anteroinferior one-third of the middle turbinate, preserving the upper two-thirds. The contact technique is used to cut the thin lamellar bone, as shown here. This results in satisfactory visualization of the surgical field without unduly disturbing the middle turbinate.

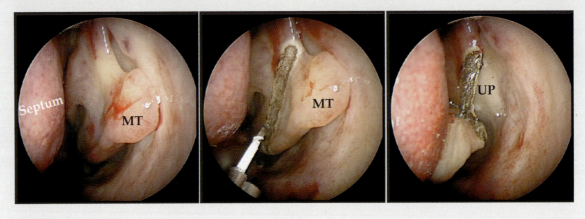

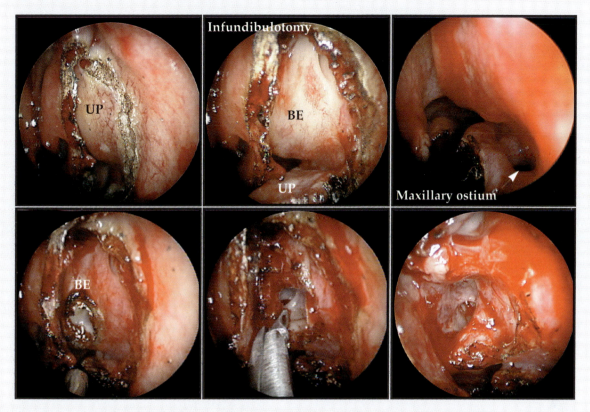

The uncinate plate is defined and a laser incision is made for a subtotal uncinectomy. The incision starts just below the upper attachment of the uncinate plate and goes inferiorly. The upper attachment of the uncinate plate is kept intact, as it serves as a landmark for the frontal recess.

The uncinate process is reflected medially and inferiorly, exposing the ethmoid infundibulum. The submucosal removal of the uncinate plate at the level of the maxillary ostium widens the ostium.

The anteroinferior wall of the bulla is resected with the laser in the near-contact mode. The medial bullar wall is resected with Thru-Cut forceps. The dissection continues until the suprabullar space is reached. The osteoma is attached to the lamina cribrosa and the fovea of the anterior ethmoid. The posterior fovea should first be clearly identified before the resection. This is done so that the lesion can be approached from behind with the micro-curette. The posterior ethmoid is entered through the oblique part of the lamella, as described previously.

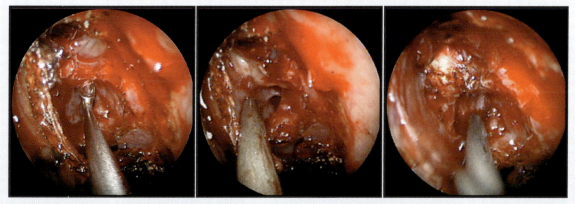

After the posterior fovea is identified, neurosurgical cottonoids soaked in oxymetazoline are placed on it. The mucosa over and at the periphery of the osteoma is lased with the KTP laser at 5 watts of power in a near-contact mode to obtain a coagulative effect. The osteoma is now delineated. The anterior ethmoid artery is located just posterosuperior to the osteoma.

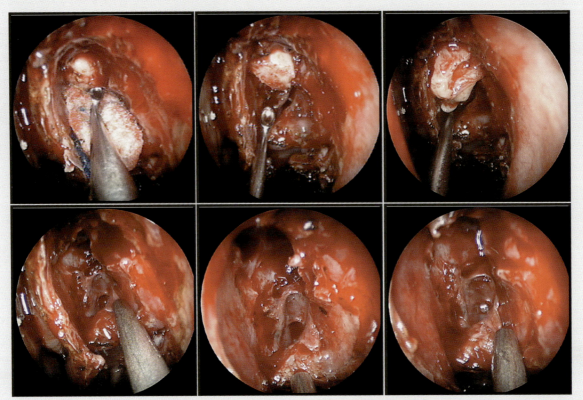

Next, the periphery of the osteoma is gently curetted with the angled microcurette. The most delicate area is the medial segment. The angled microcurette is inserted posterosuperior to the osteoma and a gentle knocking is used to dislodge it.

The surgeon should use the same precision and gentleness as in removing the stapes footplate. After dislodgment of the osteoma, the fovea and the anterior ethmoid artery are identified and inspected.

Although the risk of cerebrospinal fluid leak was anticipated and the patient was counseled about it, no such complication was encountered. The procedure was done on an outpatient basis and the postoperative course was uneventful.

This is a delicate procedure that requires a high degree of precision and accuracy. It is critical to avoid injury to surrounding structures. In my opinion, the laser serves an important role here and is of utmost value in obtaining a successful result.

Four-month postoperative axial CT sections

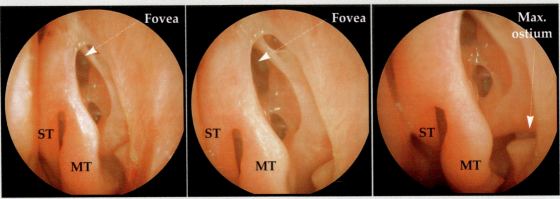

11
Computer-Guided Endoscopic Sinus Surgery

Introduction

Computer-guided surgery using the Visualization Technologies Inc. (VTI, Woburn, MA) Insta Trak electromagnetic system can decrease the potential complications of orbital or intracranial iatrogenic trauma during endoscopic sinus surgery. This device uses an electromagnetic field generator and receiving system to localize the tip of the surgical instrument during a sinus procedure.

Indications

Computer-guided surgery is especially indicated in: chronic panpolypoid rhinosinusitis, revision surgery, sphenoid sinus surgery, the presence of variant anatomy (such as an Onodi cell), tumor surgery, trauma, and whenever the surgeon feels that difficulties may be encountered during the surgical dissection.

Contraindications

None.

Surgical Technique

Following appropriate medical therapy, when surgery is planned, the patient has a preoperative axial CT scan performed with the VTI headset in position (Fig. 1). The CT data are processed by the VTI computer and the data are transferred to the operating room computer (Fig. 2).

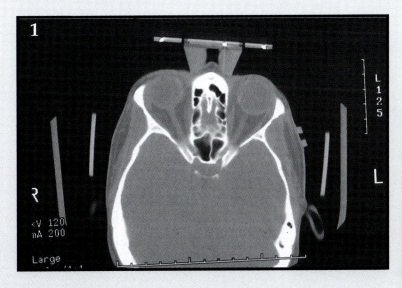

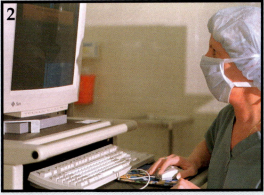

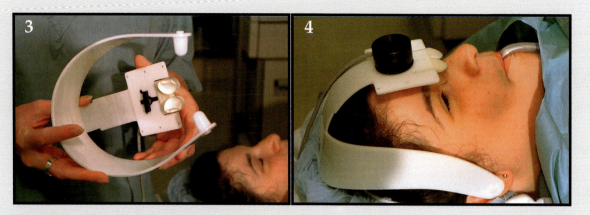

The headset (Fig. 3) is repositioned on the patient and the electromagnetic transmitter is locked into place (Fig. 4).

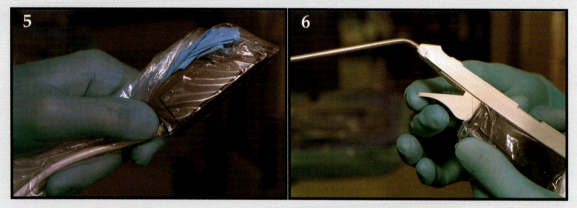

The operating field, including the headset and a separate electromagnetic receiver, are draped (Fig. 5). The receiver and attached coupler may be attached to a straight suction (Fig. 6), a curved suction, a pointer, or even to a microdebrider system.

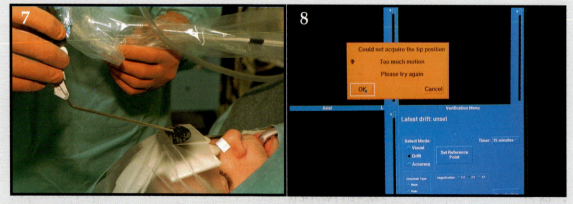

Registration, the process which allows the computer to determine the exact position of the patient on the operating table, is automatically performed by the computer. No fiducial markers are necessary. In addition, since head motion does not affect registration and tracking, surgery can be performed under either general or local anesthesia.

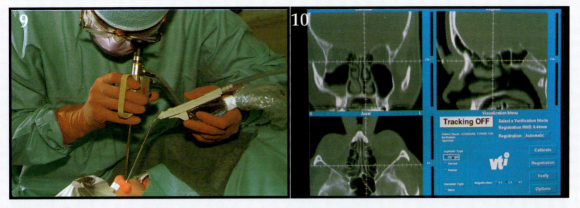

Calibration of the instrument allows the computer to take into account the lengths of the different suctions and probes. Calibration is easily performed by placing the tip of the instrument into a small dimple on the transmitter (Fig. 7) and cursoring the mouse to the appropriate menu item on the computer display. Errors, such as too much motion during the calibration, are displayed in warning boxes on the computer screen (Fig. 8). Surgery is performed paraendoscopically (Fig. 9). The location of the tip of the suction is displayed in real time as a cross hair on the axial and reconstructed coronal and parasagittal views (Fig. 10).

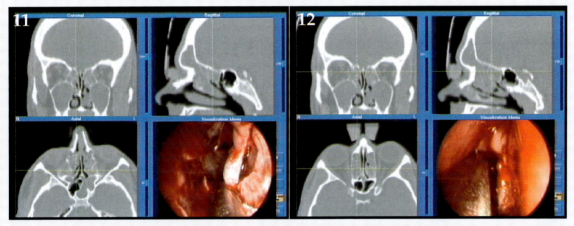

Key structures during the dissection are clearly identified with the computer:
the basal lamella (Fig. 11), the roof of the ethmoid (Fig. 12), the sphenoid sinus (Fig. 13) and the frontal recess (Fig. 14).

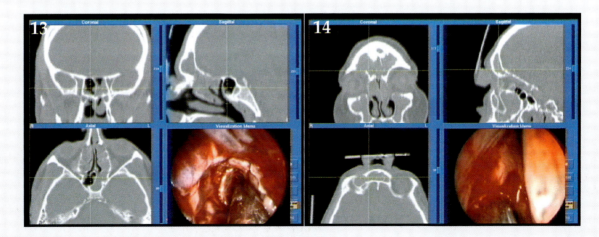

Selected References

Anon JB, Rontal M, Zinreich SJ. Anatomy of paranasal sinuses. G Thieme Verlag, 1996.

Becker, SP. Applied anatomy of the paranasal sinuses with emphasis on endoscopic surgery. Ann Otol 1994; Vol 103(Suppl 162).

Calhoun KH, Rotzler WH, Stiernburg CM. Surgical anatomy of the lateral nasal wall. Otolaryngol Head Neck Surg 1990;102:156-160.

Congdon ED. The distribution and mode of origin of septa and walls of the sphenoid sinus. Anat Rec 18, 1920.

Dixon FW. A comparative study of the sphenoid sinus (a study of 16 skulls). Ann Otol 1937;46:687-698.

Draf W. Endonasal micro-endoscopic frontal sinus surgery: The fulda concept. Operative techniques in otolaryngol 2, 1991;234-240.

Draf W. Endoscopy of the paranasal sinuses. Berlin: Springer Verlag, 1983.

Kasper KA. Nasofrontal connections: A study based on one hundred consecutive dissections. Arch Otolaryngol 23, 1936.

Lang J. Clinical anatomy of the nose, nasal cavity & paranasal sinuses. New York: G Thieme Verlag, 1989.

Mattox DE, Delaney RG. Anatomy of the ethmoid sinus. Otolaryngol Clin North Am 1985;18:3-14.

Myerson MC. The natural orifice of the maxillary sinus. Arch Otolaryng 15, 1932.

Mehta D. Atlas of endoscopic sinonasal surgery. Lea & Febiger, 1993.

Peele JC. Unusual anatomical variations of the sphenoid sinuses. Laryngoscope 1957;67:208-237.

Rice DH, Schaefer SD. Endoscopic paranasal sinus surgery. New York: Raven Press, 1993.

Ritter FN. The paranasal sinuses: anatomy and surgical technique. St. Louis: CV Mosby, 1978.

Rosenberger HC. The clinical availability of the ostium maxillare: A clinical and cadaver study. Ann Otol 47, 1938.

Rosenberger HC. Growth and development of the naso-respiratory area in childhood. Ann Otol 1934.

Schaeffer JP. The nose, paranasal sinuses, nasolacrimal passageways and olfactory organ in man. Philadelphia: Blackston, 1920;125-129.

Sethi DS, Pillay, PK. Endoscopic management of lesions of sella turcica. Journal of laryngol and otol 109, 1995;956-962.

Sethi DS, Pillay, PK. Endoscopic pituitary surgery-a minimally invasive technique. Amer journal of rhin 10,1996;141-147.

Simon E. Anatomy of the opening of the maxillary sinus ostia. Arch Otolaryngol 1939;29:640-649.

Stammberger H. Essentials of Endoscopic Sinus Surgery. Mosby-Year Book, Inc., 1993.

Stammberger HR, Kennedy DW. Paranasal sinuses: Anatomic terminology and nomenclature. Presented at International conference on sinus disease: Terminology, staging and therapy; New Jersey, 1993.

Stankiewicz JA. Advanced endoscopic sinus surgery. Mosby-Year Book, Inc., 1995.

Van Alyea DE. Ethmoid labyrinth: anatomic study with consideration of the clinical significance of its structural characteristics. Arch Otolaryngol Head Neck Surg 1939;29:881-901.

Van Alyea OE. Nasal sinuses: an anatomic and clinical consideration, 2nd ed. Baltimore: Williams & Wilkins, 1951.

Wigand ME. Endoscopic surgery of the paranasal sinuses and anterior skull base. New York: Thieme Medical Publishers, 1990;41.

Wigand ME. Endoscopic surgery of the paranasal sinuses and anterior skull base. New York: Thieme Medical Publishers, 1990.

Zinreich S, Kennedy DW, Galyler BW. Computed tomography of nasal cavity and paranasal sinuses: an evaluation of anatomy for endoscopic sinus surgery. Clear Images 1988;1:2-10.

Zuckerkandl E. Normal and Pathologische Anatomie der Nasenhohle und iher pneumatischen Anhange. Braumuller Thien. 1882;134-135.

Index

A

Accessory ostia 36, 98, 99, 104
Adjuvant procedures 148-166
  endoscopic pituitary surgery 148-153
    contraindications for 148
    indications for 148
    MRI anatomy and tumor in 149
    surgical anatomy of 48-51
    technique for endoscopic transseptal
      transsphenoidal hypophysectomy in 150-153
Agger nasi
  anatomy of 2, 3, 25, 26, 33, 42, 45-47
  bulge of 2, 8, 11, 14
  CT scan of 2, 3, 5, 8, 9, 14, 15, 25, 26, 100
  exposure of 57
  frontal sinus and 3, 16, 17, 33, 44, 57, 163
  lacrimal sac and 158
  resection of 15-17, 45, 107-109
Allergy investigation 70, 140
Anatomical variants
  in CT scan 9, 15, 35, 40, 41, 74, 76, 80, 81
  of infundibulum 40, 41
  middle meatus obstructive syndrome as
    (MMOS) 74-76
  of turbinates 70
Anatomy
  of agger nasi 2, 3, 25, 26, 33, 42, 45-47
  of basal lamella 32, 34
  of bulla ethmoidalis (ethmoid bulla) 8, 33
  of concha bullosa 34
  CT study of 2-6, 8-10, 13-15, 19, 21, 22, 24
  of ethmoid sinus 26, 30-35
  of fovea ethmoidalis 5, 10, 21, 31, 35
  of frontal sinus 3, 42-45
  of hiatus semilunaris 32, 33, 45
  of infundibulum 26, 38, 40, 105, 41, 32
  of maxillary sinus 36, 37
  of ostiomeatal unit (OMU) 10
  of pituitary 48-51, 148

  of sphenoid sinus 48-51
  of turbinates 30, 70
  of uncinate process 32, 38, 146
Anesthesia
  in dacryocystorhinostomy 158
  in ESS 88, 100
Anterior ethmoid artery 11, 18, 35, 42, 63, 106,
  165, 166
Antrostomy
  inferior meatal 102-104
  middle meatal 84-88
  nasoantral window and 102-104
Ascending process of the maxilla 8-10, 42, 106-108
  resection of 111, 112, 115, 154, 155, 158

B

Basal lamella (ground lamella)
  anatomy of 6, 32, 34
  CT scan of 15, 21, 131
  endoscopic view of 19
  injury of 19
  site of perforation of 20
  surgical technique 19-21, 116, 122, 124, 128, 129,
    132, 137, 147, 165
Basic secretion test 157
Bulla ethmoidalis (ethmoid bulla)
  anatomy of 8, 33
  approach to 11, 122
  defining boundaries of 12, 33
  in endoscopic sinus surgery (ESS) 11, 12, 85
  hypoplastic 5, 10, 11
  pneumatic 5, 7, 10, 70, 74, 76
  resection of 12, 13, 123, 124, 137, 144, 147
  shelf (floor) of 13, 15, 116
  sinus lateralis and cells of 13
  suprabullar cells of 4, 13, 33

C

Caldwell-Luc 52, 90, 140
Canaliculus
   common 154, 155, 157
   intubation of 154, 156, 157, 159-161
   lower 154
   upper 154
Canthal ligament, medial 3
Cavernous sinus 29, 49, 51
Computed tomography (CT scan)
   advantages of 24
   anatomical correlation with coronal images 24-29
   anatomical variants and 40, 41
   anatomy and 2-6, 8-10, 13-15, 19, 21, 22, 24
   axial images in 24, 63, 114, 115, 130, 142, 164, 167, 169
   of concha bullosa 82, 84
   coronal images in 2, 4, 6, 8-10, 13, 14, 19, 21, 22, 24, 156
   coronal-sectional anatomy with correlation in 24
   ethmoid series in 24
   full sinus study in 24
   of infundibulum 26, 38, 40, 41, 142
   of ostiomeatal unit (OMU) 10, 40, 41, 74, 78, 80, 82, 84, 87, 96, 98, 104, 110, 113, 120, 131, 136, 142, 144, 156, 164
   sagittal images in 3, 14, 15, 24
   sagittal reconstruction in 3, 14, 15, 24, 107
   screening study in 24
Computer-guided endoscopic sinus surgery (ESS)
   contraindications for 167
   indications for 167
   introduction to 167
   surgical technique 167-169
Concha bullosa 34, 77
   anatomy of 34
   CT scan of 82, 84
   in ESS 77, 82-84
   ethmoid sinusitis and 82, 84
   maxillary sinusitis and 82, 84
Conchal cell 6, 7, 21, 82, 83
Conchoplasty 77, 82, 83, 140
Cribriform plate 8, 10, 18, 26, 31, 81
CSF rhinorrhea 8, 18, 81

D

Dacryocystitis 155
Dacryocystogram 156, 157
Dacryocystorhinostomy, endoscopic, 154-161
   complications of 160
   concepts in 155
   dacryocystogram 156, 157
   diagnostic probing in 157
   diagnostic tests and radiological identification of lacrimal sac 156, 157
   history taking and 155
   indications for 155
   instruments and materials in 57, 156
   Jones primary dye test 157
      secondary dye test 157
   Schirmer test I and 157
   Schirmer test II and 157
   surgical technique, primary 158, 159
      anesthesia for 158
      postoperative care for 159
   surgical technique, revision-formal procedure 161
   surgical technique, revision-office procedure 160

E

Endonasal approach to frontal sinus 106-113
   revision surgery of 114-119
Endoscopic sinus surgery, (ESS) 8-23
   computer use in 167-169
   CT scan use in 1, 24, 54
   landmarks in 32-35
   minimally invasive techniques (MIT) in 52-55
Endoscopic transseptal transsphenoidal hypophysectomy 150-153
Equipment (see Surgical Instruments)
Ethmoid bulla (see Bulla Ethmoidalis)
Ethmoid infundibulum (see Ethmoid Sinus, infundibulum of)
Ethmoid sinus
   agger nasi cell and 33
   anatomy of 26, 30-35
   anterior ethmoid artery and 35
   basal lamella (ground lamella) and 32, 34
   characteristics of 31
   concha bullosa and 34
   CT scan of 19, 24-27, 35
   development of 31
   dimensions of 31

ethmoid bulla and 33
fovea ethmoidalis (see roof)
frontal bone and 30, 31, 34, 35
hiatus semilunaris inferior (Zuckerkandl), superior and 32
infraorbital ethmoid cell (Haller's cell) of 33
infundibulum of 9, 10, 32, 38
interlamellar cell and 34
lamina papyracea and 31, 33
mucosal thickening in 54, 74, 78
nasal fontanelles and 34
optic nerve tubercle and 34
pneumatization and growth of 31
posterior ethmoid and 34
posterior ethmoid artery and 35
properties of 31
roof of 5, 10, 21, 31, 35
sinusitis and 82, 84
size, adult, of 31
sphenoethmoid cell and 34
suprabullar and retrobullar recess (sinus lateralis) of 33
supraorbital ethmoid cells and 34
surgical significance 31
uncinate process and 32
Ethmoidectomy 114, 120
  anterior 110
  posterior 116, 122, 130-135
  sphenoid sinus after 126, 128, 129, 136, 137
  total 23

F

Fovea ethmoidalis (see Ethmoid Sinus, roof of)
Frontal cell (frontal bulla) 3, 30, 46, 53, 141
Frontal ostium 11, 17, 42, 44, 63, 109, 118-120
  entrance to 45-47
  location of 45-47
Frontal process of maxilla (see Ascending Process of Maxilla)
Frontal recess
  anatomy of 45
  boundaries of 47
  resection of agger nasi cell and exposure of 16
Frontal sinus
  agenesis of 43
  agger nasi and 3, 16, 17, 33, 44, 57, 163
  anatomy of 3, 42-45
  bipartite 109
  chambers of 43
  characteristics of 43
  CT scan of 59, 100, 105, 110, 119, 120
  development of 43
  dimensions of 43
  direct middle meatus course and 47
  drainage of 44, 46, 47, 106
  endonasal approach to 106-109
    principles and techniques 106
    surgical technique 106-109
  entrance into hiatus semilunaris and 47
  in ESS 110-113
  frontal cells (frontal bulla) and 46
  frontal recess and 45
  frontoethmoid disease (Group III A) and 110
    surgical technique for 110-113
  Group III A 55, 110-113, 126, 127, 138, 139
  Group III B 55, 114-137
  landmarks for revision surgery of 114
  obstruction of 110, 114, 120
  orbital recess course and 46
  ostia of 11, 17, 42, 44, 63, 109, 118-120
  pansinusitis with polyposis (Group III B) and 120-125
    KTP laser use for 123-125
    microdebrider use for 121-123
    surgical technique for 120-125
  pneumatization and growth of 43
  revision endonasal surgery (Group III B) of 114
    landmarks for 114
    surgical technique for 114-119
  size, adult, of 43
  surgical significance 43
  uncinate process and 42
Frontoethmoid disease 110-113
  KTP laser use and 110-112
  landmarks of 106
  microdebrider use and 62, 121-123
  pansinusitis and 120, 121
  polyposis and 120, 121
  power drill use and 57, 62, 112
  revision surgery of 114-119

G

Graves' ophthalmopathy 162
Ground lamella (see Basal Lamella)

H

Haller's cell 30, 33, 40, 41, 80, 163
Headache
  rhinogenic of 75
Hiatus semilunaris
  anatomy of 32, 33, 45
  depth of 38
  drainage into 44, 45, 47
  entrance, superior-lateral, into 47
  lateralized concha and 75
  uncinate process and 38

I

Image guided sinus surgery
  (see Computer-Guided ESS)
Infraorbital ethmoid cell (see Haller's Cell)
Infundibulotomy 10, 98
Infundibulum
  anatomical variants of 40, 41
  anatomy of 26, 32, 38, 40, 41, 105
  CT scan of 26, 38, 40, 41, 142
  ethmoid 9, 10, 32, 38
  Nick's Triangle and 39, 41, 121
  surgical significance of 41
  two ostia in 98-99
Instruments (see Surgical Instruments)
Internal carotid artery 29, 34
  injury of 27, 49, 127
  pituitary and 50, 148
  sphenoid sinus and 28, 49-51, 127, 138, 151

J

Jones primary dye test 157

L

Lacrimal
  bone, resection of 154, 155, 159, 161
  duct, naso- 36, 154, 155
  duct, naso-, CT scan of 25
  fossa 3, 159
  fossa, naso-, CT scan of 8
  sac 25, 106, 108, 109, 154-161
  sac, CT scan of 110, 113, 136, 156
Lamina cribrosa 7, 8, 17, 35
Lasers 66-69
  absorbing chromophore comparison of 67
  absorption length comparison of 67
  active medium comparison of 67
  application of systems in endoscopic
    sinus surgery 67
  Argon 66, 67, 69
  CO_2 66, 67, 69
  color spectrum of 67
  comparative study of 67
  excitation source comparison of 67
  Holmium (Ho:YAG) 66, 67, 69
  KTP/532 66-69
  light interaction and 69
  ND:YAG 66, 67, 69
  power range comparison of 67
  relative scatter of laser light comparison of 69
  setup for 68
  surgical dosage v. tissue effect and 69
  surgical effect v. contact mode and 69
  tissue interactions and 69
  wavelength comparison of 67
  zones of lateral thermal damage and 69
Light pipe 44, 156, 158

M

Maxillary endoscopy
  biopsy and 88, 90
  canine fossa and 88, 92, 98
    ostiomeatal unit obstruction and 104, 105
  contraindications for 88
  dye study and 90-92, 98, 99, 104
  in ESS 91-94, 98, 99, 104
  indications for 88
  surgical technique 88-94
  techniques of biopsy and excision of polyps and
    cysts and 90-94
Maxillary ostium 32, 36, 38-40, 90, 91, 93, 104, 105, 143, 146
  access to 38
  anatomy of 38
  location of 36, 39, 40
  reconstruction of 60, 84-87, 95-97, 100-102, 121, 123, 162
    with microdebrider 95-97
Maxillary sinus
  accessory ostium and 36
  agenesis of 37

anatomy of 36, 37
anterior wall and 36
capacity of 37
chambers of 37
characteristics of 37
CT scan of 88, 101, 105
development of 37
dimensions of 37
in ESS 10, 38, 39, 60, 78, 82, 84-87
floor of 36
infundibular anatomical variations on
   CT scan and 40, 41
isolated lesions in 91
management of chronic sinusitis and 100-102
mucosal thickening in 92, 101, 105
nasolacrimal duct and 36
Nick's Triangle and 39, 41
obstruction of 82, 84, 101, 142, 144
pneumatization and growth of 37
posterior wall and 36
roof of 36
sinusitis and 100
size, adult, of 37
surgical significance 37, 41
Microdebrider 57-59, 66, 77, 95, 97, 125, 141, 168
   advantages of 56, 58, 59
   Apex Shaver System 57, 58
   ESSential Sinus Shaver 58
   Hummer-ENT Microdebrider 58
   surgical technique 59-65, 95-97, 121-123
   XPS Straightshot Micro Resector System 57, 59, 95
Middle meatal antrostomy 84-88
Middle meatus obstructive syndrome (MMOS) 74
   anatomical variants and 74
   in ESS 74-83
Middle meatus reconstruction (MMR) 74
   concha bullosa and 77
   conchoplasty and 82, 83
      surgical technique of 74
   hypertrophic concha and 75
   large pneumatic bulla ethmoidalis and 76
   large pneumatic uncinate process and 76
   lateralized concha and 75
   middle turbinoplasty and 78, 79
      advantages of 78
      surgical technique of 79
   middle turbinotomy and 74
   paradoxical concha and 81

partial conchal resection and 77
surgical technique 74-83
Minimally invasive techniques (MIT)
   in ESS 52-55
   instruments in 56, 57
   lasers in 66-69
   microdebrider in 58-65
   in pediatric sinus disease 140-147
   principles of 54, 55
   surgical technique with microdebrider 59-65
MRI anatomy and pituitary tumor 149

N

Nasal congestion and obstruction 54, 70, 74, 84, 100, 110, 142
Nasion 3
   CT scan and 2, 9, 17, 24, 25, 59-61, 64, 65, 113, 136
Nasoantral window 52
   connection to natural ostium 103
   surgical technique 102-105
Nick's Triangle 39, 41, 121, 145
   approach to infundibulum and 39, 41

O

Onodi cells 6, 7, 30, 34, 129
Optic nerve
   ethmoid cells and 26, 27
   injury of 6, 22, 27, 127, 129
   orbital decompression and 162
   sphenoid sinus and 22, 27, 28, 50, 103, 130, 138
   tubercle 34
Orbital decompression
   frontal recess in 163
   Haller's cell in 163
   indications for 162
   maxillary ostium in 162
   pathology of 162
   surgical technique 162, 163
Orbital injury 9-11
Osteoma
   surgical technique for 164-166
Ostiomeatal unit (OMU)
   anatomy of 10
   CT scan of 10, 40, 41, 74, 78, 80, 82, 84, 87, 96, 98, 104, 110, 113, 120, 131, 136, 142, 144, 156, 164

maxillary endoscopy and 88
maxillary ostium reconstruction and 84-87
middle meatal antrostomy and 84-87
obstruction of 81, 84-87, 92, 94, 101
canine fossa maxillary endoscopy and 104, 105
inferior meatal antrostomy and 102-104
and management of chronic maxillary
   sinusitis 100-102
nasoantral window and 102-104
and two ostia in infundibulum 98-99
sinusitis and 74, 78, 80-82, 84
surgical technique for reconstruction of,
   with KTP laser 84-87
   with microdebrider 95-97

P

Pansinusitis
  with polyposis 120-125, 136, 137
Paranasal sinuses, (see specific sinus)
Pediatric sinus disease
  algorithm of sinusitis in 140
  conservative treatment of 140
  CT scan in 141, 142, 144
  ESS in 143-147
  investigations for 140
  minimally invasive techniques (MIT) in 140-147
  polypectomy in 142, 143
  principles of minimally invasive techniques
    (MIT) in 140
  surgical management of 140
  turbinoplasty in 145
Pituitary
  anatomy of 148
  cavernous sinus and 29
  contraindications for surgery of 148
  endoscopic transseptal transsphenoidal
    hypophysectomy 150-153
  indications for surgery of 148
  internal carotid artery and 148
  optic chiasma and 149
  optic nerve and 50
  sphenoid sinus and 148
  surgical technique 150-153
Pneumatization (see specific sinus)
Polyposis 120-125, 136, 137
Polyps 88, 90-92, 94, 139, 142, 143
Posterior ethmoid artery 22, 35, 42

Posterior ethmoid, in ESS 20-22, 134

R

Radiography (see Computed Tomography)
Rhinopathy
  chronic 70
  types of 70

S

Sella turcica 28, 29, 151
Sinus cells (see specific sinus)
Sinus disease
  algorithm of 55
  Group I 55, 70-73
  Group II 55, 84-87
  Group III A 55, 110-113, 126, 127, 138, 139
  Group III B 55, 114-137
Sinusitis 52, 53, 55, 75, 82, 94, 96, 100, 110, 114,
  130, 138, 140, 142, 144, 157, 164, 167
  CT scan and 52-55, 74, 78, 80, 82, 84, 87-88, 93,
    96, 98, 100, 105, 113-115, 119, 120, 130, 131,
    136, 142, 144, 167
  endoscopic sinus surgery (ESS) and 11, 125
  maxillary sinus and 10, 11, 13, 19, 82, 86-92,
    99-103, 105, 123, 142, 146
  patient history and 52-55
Sphenoid sinus
  agenesis of 49
  anatomy of 48-51
  carotid artery and 28, 49-51, 127, 138, 151
  chambers of 49
  characteristics of 48, 49
  CT scan and 15, 22, 24, 27, 28, 63, 102, 103,
    129, 130
  development of 49
  dimensions of 49
  drainage of 130, 138
  ESS and 22, 169
  ethmoid and 30, 31
  ethmoidectomy, posterior and 130-135
  intrasphenoid projections 50
  isolated disease of 126
  obstruction of 127, 130
  optic nerve and 22, 27, 28, 34, 50, 103, 129,
    130, 138
  ostium of 15, 48, 50

pansinusitis with polyposis
(Group III B) and 136, 137
surgical technique 136, 137
pituitary and 148
pneumatization and growth of 49
pneumatization, types of 48
recess, sphenoethmoid 51, 136, 138
recess, supraoptic and infraoptic of 50
rostrum 28, 51, 129, 138, 139, 150-152
size, adult, of 49
sphenoethmoidal recess of 51, 136, 138
sphenoethmoidectomy (Group III B),
technique for, 128, 129
sphenoidotomy (Group III B),
technique for, 130-135
revision (Group III A) 138
surgical technique for revision
(Group III A) 138, 139
surgical significance of 49
surgical technique for isolated disease
(Group III A) of 126, 127
transethmoid approach to 22
Sphenoidotomy 126-127, 130-135, 137, 150-151
carotid artery and 138
revision 138, 139
Surgical instruments 56, 57
(also see Lasers)
(also see Microdebrider)
Power drill (Fisch drill) 57, 62, 106, 108, 115, 155

T
Tooth
canine 36, 88, 92, 93
in ESS 92
in maxillary sinus 92, 93
Turbinates
adjunct to ESS 70
adjunct to septal surgery 70
anatomical variants and 70
anatomy of 30, 70
CT scan of 3-6, 19, 21, 72, 74, 78, 80, 81, 101, 110
dysfunction of 70
hypertrophic concha 70, 74, 75
indications for surgery of 70
inferior 30
techniques for surgery of 71-73
laser turbinotomy 100, 110, 164

advantages of 73
submucous 73
lateralized concha 75, 80
middle 30
conchoplasty and 82, 83
lateralized 70, 110
partial conchal resection of 70, 77, 100, 110,
126, 132, 164
stability of 23
turbinotomy 74
mucosal contact of 70
multiple island technique 71, 72
objective in surgery of 71
paradoxical concha 81, 100
stripes with cross-hatching technique 72
superior 30
supreme 30
surgical indications for 70
surgical objective 71
surgical technique 70-83
turbinoplasty 78-79, 145
advantages of 78

U
Uncinate process 4, 5, 9, 26, 32, 38, 40-42, 84
anatomy of 32, 38, 146
course of 5
in ESS 59-62, 85, 165
frontal sinus and 42
pneumatic 9, 70, 76
Uncinectomy 10, 11, 95
microdebrider use and 95-97
partial, in ESS, 38, 39, 84-87, 100, 101, 105,
145, 146
subtotal, in ESS, 111, 123, 165

Endoscopic Sinus Surgery
New Horizons
Interactive CD-ROM
Nikhil J. Bhatt, M.D.

The first true interactive multimedia presentation prepared in its entirety by a surgeon!

This **CD-ROM** is designed to sharpen the technical knowledge of the endoscopic sinus surgeon. Nasal and paranasal sinus pathology in adults and children is demonstrated along with diagnostic criteria and specific treatments. Application of this knowledge will result in safer techniques and more successful outcomes.

This multimedia presentation has been formatted in a way that allows the viewer to select and study the specific parts that interest him or her.

The CD-ROM contains narrated video clips on minimally invasive techniques for anatomical variants, ostiomeatal unit disease, endonasal approach to the frontal sinus, and sphenoid sinus diseases, which provides a panorama of educational material.

❏ **Interactive CD-ROM Volume 1**
- Surgical Significance of the Anatomical Landmarks and Surgical Techniques
- Coronal-Sectional Anatomy with CT Section Correlations
- Regional Surgical Anatomy
- Minimally Invasive Techniques in Endoscopic Sinus Surgery
- Microdebriders and Lasers
- Surgical Techniques for Turbinates and Anatomical Variants
- Surgical Techniques for Ostiomeatal Unit Obstruction

❏ **Interactive CD-ROM Volume 2**
- Endonasal Approach to the Frontal Sinus
- Sphenoid Sinus Surgery
- Minimally Invasive Techniques in Pediatric Sinus Diseases
- Adjuvant Procedures
  Endoscopic Pituitary Surgery
  Dacryocystorhinostomy—Primary and Revision
  Orbital Decompression
  Osteoma
- Computer-Guided Endoscopic Sinus Surgery

Minimally Invasive Surgical Techniques
companion videos to
Endoscopic Sinus Surgery: New Horizons
Nikhil J. Bhatt, M.D.

An excellent resource for the surgeon without CD-ROM capabilities!

These companion videos on minimally invasive techniques for anatomical variants, ostiomeatal unit disease, endonasal approach to the frontal sinus, and sphenoid sinus diseases provide a panorama of educational material.

The companion videos on minimally invasive techniques provide full frame live surgical procedures covered in the **Endoscopic Sinus Surgery: New Horizons** book and CD-ROM.

PAL & NTSC formats are available.

❏ **Volume 1 • Laser Surgical Techniques**
- Turbinate Reduction and Turbinotomy
- Conchoplasty and Turbinoplasty
- Middle Meatus Reconstruction with Partial Middle Turbinotomy
- Partial Uncinectomy and Infundibulotomy with Maxillary Ostium Reconstruction
- Anterior Ethmoidectomy and Bulla and Suprabullar Cell Resection
- Frontal Recess and Frontal Ostium Reconstruction
- Revision Surgery
- Sphenoidotomy
- Sphenoethmoidectomy
- Pediatric Sinus Surgery
- Dacryocystorhinostomy

❏ **Volume 2 • Microdebrider Surgical Techniques**
- Inferior Turbinotomy - Reduction
- Middle Meatus Reconstruction with Partial Middle Turbinotomy
- Partial Excision of Concha Bullosa
- Partial Uncinectomy and Infundibulotomy with Maxillary Ostium Reconstruction
- Total Uncinectomy and Agger Cell Resection
- Anterior Ethmoidectomy and Bulla and Suprabullar Cell Resection
- Basal Lamella and Posterior Ethmoidectomy
- Sphenoidotomy
- Frontal Recess and Frontal Ostium Reconstruction
- Dacryocystorhinostomy

SINGULAR PUBLISHING GROUP
CALL TOLL FREE 1-800-521-8545

TOLL FREE FAX ORDER FORM
FAX TOLL FREE 1-800-774-8398

ORDERED BY
Name _____
Inst./Co. _____
Address _____
City _____
State _____ Zip _____
Day Phone Number _____
(Required with all orders)

DELIVER TO (only if different than ordered by)
Name _____
Inst./Co. _____
Address _____
City _____
State _____ Zip _____
**UPS CANNOT DELIVER TO A P.O. BOX
PLEASE PROVIDE A STREET ADDRESS**

SHIPPING OPTIONS (Please check one)

- ❏ UPS Ground Service $6.00 first item, $2.25 each add'l
- ❏ UPS 3rd Day Air $10.00 first item, $3.50 each add'l
- ❏ UPS 2nd Day Air $14.75 first item, $4.00 each add'l
- ❏ UPS Next Day Air $24.00 first item, $7.75 each add'l
- ❏ Foreign Book Rate: $ same as UPS Ground Service
- ❏ Foreign Air Mail: same as UPS Next Day

METHOD OF PAYMENT

- ❏ MasterCard   ❏ Visa
- ❏ American Express   ❏ Discover
- ❏ Check*   ❏ P.O. Enclosed

*Payable in U.S. currency drawn on a U.S. bank.

Name of Cardholder _____   Signature _____
Credit Card Number _____   Exp. Date _____

Endoscopic Sinus Surgery
New Horizons

Title	Code	Price	Quantity	Total
CD-ROM Value Pack (includes book and CD-ROM Volumes I & II)	1780	$295.00	_____	_____
Interactive CD-ROM Volumes I & II	1772	$175.00	_____	_____
Video Volume I - Lasers*	1774	$99.00	_____	_____
Video Volume II - Microdebriders*	1776	$99.00	_____	_____
Video Volumes I & II**	1778	$175.00	_____	_____
Video Value Pack** (includes book and video Volumes I & II)	1782	$275.00	_____	_____
Combo Value Pack** (includes book, CD-ROM and video Volumes I & II)	1784	$395.00	_____	_____
Endoscopic Sinus surgery (book)	1766	$129.00	_____	_____

Circle one: * Add $50.00 for PAL format
NTSC/PAL   ** Add $75.00 for PAL format

Subtotal _____
CA residents add CA sales tax _____
Shipping and Handling _____
TOTAL _____

Return Policy: If a book does not meet your expectations, you may return it in resalable condition within 30 days of purchase for a refund of the purchase price less our shipping cost. No refunds on software or videotape purchases. Defective tapes or disks will be replaced.
Prices are subject to change without notice.

Mail to: **SINGULAR PUBLISHING GROUP, INC.** • 401 WEST "A" STREET, SUITE 325 • SAN DIEGO, CA 92101-7904

E-Mail: singpub@mail.cerfnet.com   Website: http://www.singpub.com